Biofunctional Scaffolds for Spinal Cord Regeneration
Jerani T. S. Pettikiriarachchi, Malcolm K. Horne, John S. Forsythe, and David R. Nisbet
2010. ISBN: 978-1-61668-757-1

Biofunctional Scaffolds for Spinal Cord Regeneration
Jerani T. S. Pettikiriarachchi, Malcolm K. Horne, John S. Forsythe, and David R. Nisbet
2010. ISBN: 978-1-61728-256-0
(E-book)

Infectious Disease Modelling Research Progress
Jean Michel Tchuenche and C. Chiyaka (Editors)
2010. ISBN: 978-1-60741-347-9

Home Fire Safety: Preventive Measures and Issues
Cornelio Moretti (Editor)
2009. ISBN: 978-1-60741-651-7

Expedited Partner Therapy in the Management of STDs
H. Hunter Handsfield, Matthew Hogben, Julia A. Schillinger, Matthew R. Golden, Patricia Kissinger and P. Frederick Sparling
2010. ISBN: 978-1-60741-571-8

Periodontitis: Symptoms, Treatment and Prevention
Rosemarie E. Walchuck (Editor
2010. ISBN: 978-1-61668-836-3

Periodontitis: Symptoms, Treatment and Prevention
Rosemarie E. Walchuck (Editor
2010. ISBN: 978-1-61728-072-6
(E-book)

EMS Workforce for the 21st Century - A National Assessment
Javier C. Bailey (Editor
2010. ISBN: 978-1-60741-998-3

Handbook of Disease Outbreaks: Prevention, Detection and Control
Albin Holmgren and Gerhard Borg (Editors)
2010. ISBN: 978-1-60876-224-8

Overweightness and Walking
Caleb I. Black (Editor)
2010. ISBN: 978-1-60741-298-4

Overweightness and Walking
Caleb I. Black (Editor)
2010. ISBN: 978-1-61668-516-4
(E-book)

Smoking Relapse: Causes, Prevention and Recovery
Johan Egger and Mikel Kalb (Editors)
2010. ISBN: 978-1-60876-580-5

Medicare Advantage: The Alternate Medicare Program
Charles V. Baylis (Editors)
2010. ISBN: 978-1-60876-031-2

PUBLIC HEALTH IN THE 21ST CENTURY

THE ANTI-INFLAMMATORY EFFECTS OF EXERCISE

PUBLIC HEALTH IN THE 21ST CENTURY

PUBLIC HEALTH IN THE 21ST CENTURY

THE ANTI-INFLAMMATORY EFFECTS OF EXERCISE

PEDRO TAULER
AND
ANTONI AGUILÓ

Nova Science Publishers, Inc.

New York

NOTICE TO THE READER

The Publisher has taken reasonable care in the preparation of this book, but makes no expressed or implied warranty of any kind and assumes no responsibility for any errors or omissions. No liability is assumed for incidental or consequential damages in connection with or arising out of information contained in this book. The Publisher shall not be liable for any special, consequential, or exemplary damages resulting, in whole or in part, from the readers' use of, or reliance upon, this material.

Independent verification should be sought for any data, advice or recommendations contained in this book. In addition, no responsibility is assumed by the publisher for any injury and/or damage to persons or property arising from any methods, products, instructions, ideas or otherwise contained in this publication.

This publication is designed to provide accurate and authoritative information with regard to the subject matter covered herein. It is sold with the clear understanding that the Publisher is not engaged in rendering legal or any other professional services. If legal or any other expert assistance is required, the services of a competent person should be sought. FROM A DECLARATION OF PARTICIPANTS JOINTLY ADOPTED BY A COMMITTEE OF THE AMERICAN BAR ASSOCIATION AND A COMMITTEE OF PUBLISHERS.

LIBRARY OF CONGRESS CATALOGING-IN-PUBLICATION DATA

Tauler, Pedro.
  The anti-inflammatory effects of exercise / authors, Pedro Tauler, Antoni Aguiló.
    p. ; cm.
  Includes bibliographical references and index.
  ISBN 978-1-60876-886-8 (softcover)
  1. Inflammation. 2. Exercise--Physiological aspects. I. Aguiló, Antoni. II. Title.
  [DNLM: 1. Exercise. 2. Inflammation--prevention & control. QZ 150 T225a 2009]
  RB131.T38 2009   616'.0473--dc22
                                                        2009050472

Published by Nova Science Publishers, Inc. ✝ *New York*

CONTENTS

Preface		xi
Chapter 1	Introduction	1
Chapter 2	Components of the Inflammatory Response	3
Chapter 3	Evidences for Inflammation in Chronic Diseases: Low-Grade Systemic Inflammation	7
Chapter 4	Acute Effects of Exercise on Immune Function	11
Chapter 5	Acute Exercise and Circulating Cytokine Levels	13
Chapter 6	Anti-Inflammatory Response Induced by Acute Exercise: Role of IL-6	17
Chapter 7	Anti-Inflammatory Effects of Chronic Moderate Exercise	23
Conclusion		31
References		33
Index		51

PREFACE

Public health recommendations concerning physical activity   state that moderate-intensity aerobic   activity for a minimum of 30 min   for at least five days   a week   may offer substantial protection against chronic diseases; such as, cardiovascular disease, atherosclerosis, type 2 diabetes, insulin resistance, colon cancer, and breast cancer. The mechanisms responsible for these protective effects by exercise are not completely clear. Nowadays it is well-known that these diseases are associated with chronic low-grade systemic inflammation. Thus, it has been suggested that the modification of the levels   for inflammation markers may have therapeutic potential.

In general, the plasma cytokines found following acute bouts of exercise suggest that exercise induces a strong anti-inflammatory effect. This finding may provide, in part, a mechanism as to why physical exercise either reduces the susceptibility to; or improves the symptoms of diseases associated with low-grade inflammation. In fact, muscle contraction induces the production of factors with anti-inflammatory properties, which are released to the circulation during exercise. These anti-inflammatory factors released by the muscle may be involved in mediating the health beneficial effects of exercise, playing important roles in the protection against these diseases associated with low-grade inflammation. Furthermore, cross-sectional studies demonstrate an association between physical inactivity and low-grade systemic inflammation in healthy subjects, in elderly people, as well as in patients with intermittent claudication. However, it is not clear how chronic moderate exercise could perform its anti-inflammatory effects. It has been hypothesized that the long-term healthy effect of exercise may, to some extent, be ascribed to the anti-inflammatory response elicited by acute bouts of moderate exercise. In addition, it has been suggested that following acute exercise, there is a transient increase in circulating levels of anti-inflammatory factors, whereas chronic exercise reduces basal levels of pro-inflammatory cytokines. Recent studies have suggested that continuous subtle changes resulting in reductions in fat and body mass or in improved lipid and glycemic profiles could induce the anti-inflammatory effect of regular moderate-intensity exercise.

The aim of this review is to examine the anti-inflammatory effects of aerobic exercise and to discuss to what extend the exercise induced anti-inflammatory response may play a therapeutic role in chronic diseases associated with low-grade inflammation.

Chapter 1

INTRODUCTION

Public health recommendations concerning physical activity state that moderate-intensity aerobic activity for a minimum of 30 min for at least five days a week may offer substantial protection against chronic diseases; such as, cardiovascular disease, type 2 diabetes and others [1, 2]. Regular physical activity was independent of body mass index (BMI) and associated with lower risk for both cardiovascular mortality and cancer mortality [3].

On the other hand, physical inactivity has been recently suggested to be a disease in itself and proposed to be the most important behavioral cause of insulin resistance [4]. In fact, physical inactivity accelerates the development of major chronic disease, with studies showing a particularly marked and consistent effect on cardiovascular disease [5]. Several studies have demonstrated a BMI–independent association between low fitness level and all-cause mortality [6-11], as well as between a low level of self-reported physical activity and premature mortality [12-20]. Moreover, physical inactivity has been identified as a stronger predictor of these chronic diseases than risk factors such as hypertension, hyperlipidemia, diabetes, and obesity for all-cause mortality [6]. It should be highlighted that chronic diseases are the largest cause of death in the world, led by cardiovascular disease followed by cancer, chronic lung diseases, and diabetes mellitus [21]. Regular exercise offers protection against all-cause mortality, primarily protection against atherosclerosis, type 2 diabetes, colon cancer, and breast cancer [21]. In fact, there is clinical general evidence for a beneficial effect of continuous moderate physical activity in patients with chronic diseases. The evidence for prescribing exercise in patients with chronic diseases was reviewed; an excellent source [22]. Randomized intervention studies have shown that physical training is effective in the treatment of patients with, among others, ischemic heart disease, insulin resistance, type 2 diabetes, dyslipemias, chronic obstructive pulmonary disease (COPD), cancer [22] and heart failure [23, 24].

Over the past decade, there has been an increased focus on the role of inflammation in the pathogenesis of atherosclerosis [25]. Furthermore, inflammation has been suggested to be a key factor in insulin resistance [26]. In this sense, the term low-grade chronic inflammation, that is characterized by increased systemic levels of some cytokines and C-reactive protein (CRP) [27], has been introduced to describe the inflammatory picture found in several chronic diseases. Some reports investigate various markers of inflammation and have confirmed an association between low-grade systemic inflammation, on one hand; and atherosclerosis and type 2 diabetes on the other [28]. Recent findings demonstrate that physical activity induces an increase in the systemic levels of a number of cytokines with anti-inflammatory properties [29] and skeletal muscle have recently been identified as an endocrine organ that produces and releases cytokines [29-32].

Given that chronic low-grade systemic inflammation may be involved in several chronic diseases and by the finding that physical exercise induces an increase in levels of some cytokines with anti-inflammatory properties; we discuss whether physical activity exerts anti-inflammatory effects; and, as a consequence, could protect against chronic diseases associated with low-grade systemic inflammation.

Chapter 2

COMPONENTS OF THE INFLAMMATORY RESPONSE

The local response to infections or tissue injury involves the production of cytokines that are released at the site of inflammation [29]. Cytokines are small polypeptides, which were originally supposed to have immuno-regulatory roles [33, 34]. Some of these cytokines facilitate an influx of lymphocytes, neutrophils, monocytes, and other cells to the site of inflammation [29]. The local inflammatory response is accompanied by a systemic response known as the acute-phase response. This response includes the production of several acute phase proteins, such as C reactive protein (CRP), produced by the liver, and can be mimicked by the injection of the cytokines tumor necrosis factor α (TNF-α, IL-1β, and IL-6 into laboratory animals or humans [33-35]. The initial cytokines in the cytokine cascade are, in order of appearance, TNF-α, IL-1β, IL-6, IL-1 receptor antagonist (IL-1ra), and soluble TNF-α receptors (sTNFR). IL-1ra inhibits IL-1 signal transduction and sTNF-R represents the naturally occurring inhibitor of TNF-α [33-35]. In response to an acute infection or trauma, the cytokines and cytokine inhibitors may increase several folds and decrease when the infection or trauma is healed [29]. Some of the cytokines involved in the inflammatory response are clearly pro-inflammatory (e.g. IL-1, TNF-α) but others are mainly anti-inflammatory (e.g. IL-10, IL-1ra). Whereas IL-10 influences multiple cytokines inhibiting their production [36-38], the biological role of IL-1ra is to inhibit signaling transduction through the IL-1 receptor complex [39]. In fact, both pro- and anti-inflammatory cytokines play an essential role after tissue injury or infection. For example, it has been recently suggested that during skeletal muscle regeneration an inflammatory stage followed by an anti-inflammatory one are essential in order to complete tissue regeneration [40]. Whereas the inflammatory environment stage is characterized by removing necrotic tissue, during the anti-inflammatory one the myogenic differentiation and muscle repair is produced [40].

The particularities of each cytokine will not be discussed. However, it could be interesting to highlight several aspects regarding cytokine production and its roles. As mentioned earlier, there is an interesting but also complex relation between immune system and cytokines. For example, it has been indicated that T lymphocytes can be classified as type 1 or type 2 cells, depending on which cytokines they predominantly produce [41]. Type 1 T lymphocytes produce mainly TNF-□, and their actions activate macrophages and induce killer mechanisms, including T-cytotoxic cells, thus driving the immune system toward cell-mediated immune responses, which primarily provide protection against intracellular pathogens such as viruses. Type 2 lymphocytes mainly synthesize IL-4, IL-5, IL-10, and IL-13, and are necessary for promotion of humoral immunity; IgE-mediated allergic reactions and activation of potentially tissue-damaging eosinophils. IL-4 and IL-13 primarily drive B-cell differentiation to antibody production, while IL-5 stimulates and primes eosinophils. Together with IL-4, IL-10 (which is also produced by monocytes and B cells) can inhibit type 1 T-cell cytokine production.

However, most of the recent research has been focused on IL-6 and its production in muscle. Skeletal muscle, the largest organ in the human body, has recently been identified as an endocrine organ that produces and releases cytokines [29-32]. In fact, during physical exercise IL-6 is ·predominantly produced within the working skeletal muscles [42-44]. Muscle contraction is supposed to activate this production and release cytokines, which could influence metabolism and modify cytokine production in tissue and organs as well as in immune cells. IL-6 is induced in skeletal muscle via a Ca^{2+} dependent pathway [45] and acts through AMP-activated kinase [46-48]. Due to its complex role in both metabolism and inflammation, IL-6 has been proposed as the key factor during exercise [32].

As indicated previously, the production of cytokines is influenced, among other factors, by myokine release. Furthermore, once released transiently into the blood stream, myokines mediate some of the systemic and beneficial effects of exercise in non-muscle tissue, e.g. modulation of hepatic glucose production through IL-6. Thus, the transient fluctuations of myokines following physical activity, that will be discussed later, might contribute to the beneficial effects of exercise on organs other than muscle in a hormone-like fashion; whereas chronic elevation of many of these same molecules is almost certainly pro-inflammatory and detrimental. It has been suggested that because systemic markers of inflammation are elevated in several chronic diseases, modifying their levels through exercise may have therapeutic potential [49].

Chapter 3

EVIDENCES FOR INFLAMMATION IN CHRONIC DISEASES: LOW-GRADE SYSTEMIC INFLAMMATION

Inflammation has been considered as the natural host response to an acute infectious episode, whereas chronic inflammation has been considered a sign of chronic infection. It has now become clear that low-grade chronic inflammation is a key player in the pathogenesis of most chronic diseases [50]. In this sense, the concept of low-grade chronic inflammation has been introduced and it is now widely used [29]. Low-grade chronic inflammation is characterized by increased systemic levels of some cytokines and, specially, C-reactive protein (CRP) [27]. Chronic low-grade systemic inflammation has been introduced as a term for conditions in which a two to three-fold increase in the systemic concentrations of TNF-α, IL-1, IL-6, IL-1ra, sTNF-R, and CRP is reflected [29]. In this sense, chronically elevated levels of systemic IL-6, IL-8, IL-10, IL-1, or TNF-α have been linked to the development of many diseases associated with inflammation including cancer, COPD, rheumatoid arthritis and other age-associated diseases such as sarcopenia [51-57]. In addition, chronic elevation of IL-6 and TNF-α results in skeletal muscle atrophy and inhibition of muscle regeneration, respectively [58, 59]. Furthermore, chronically elevated serum IL-6 levels have a predictive value for obesity and type 2 diabetes [60]. Plasma IL-6, TNF-α and CRP have emerged as strong independent risk factors for cardiovascular diseases development [61].

As it has been previously suggested, recent findings indicate that many chronic diseases have been found to be associated with this sterile, persistent, low-grade systemic inflammation. For example, the development of insulin resistance

[26, 62] and type 2 diabetes is closely correlated with immune cell infiltration and inflammation in white adipose tissue [51]. In cardiovascular diseases, activated immune cells and inflammation play a major role, particularly in the etiology of atherosclerosis [25, 49, 52, 63]. Furthermore, COPD is characterized by chronic inflammation, with high levels of TNF-α both in blood [55] and in the muscle [57]. Several reports investigate various markers of inflammation and have confirmed an association between low-grade systemic inflammation, on one hand; and atherosclerosis and type 2 diabetes on the other [28]. Inflammation has been also observed in rheumatoid arthritis, characterized by permanent high levels of circulating TNF-α levels [56]. Increasing evidence suggests that TNF-α plays a direct role in the metabolic syndrome [64], pointing to an effect of TNF-α on insulin signaling. TNF-α impairs insulin-stimulated rates of glucose storage in cultured human muscle cells and impairs insulin-mediated glucose uptake in rats. TNF-α protein is elevated locally and systemically in diabetes model animals [65]. Furthermore, neutralization of TNF-α in obese rats caused a significant increase in the peripheral uptake of glucose in response to insulin [65]. These results point to a role for TNF-α in the insulin resistance and diabetes that often accompany obesity. After adjustment for multiple confounders, including IL-6, high plasma TNF-α concentrations have been associated with insulin resistance [66] and evidence for a direct role of TNF-α in insulin resistance in humans *in vivo* has been obtained [64]. It was demonstrated that TNF-α infusion in healthy humans induces insulin resistance in skeletal muscle without an effect on endogenous glucose production. TNF-α directly impaired glucose uptake and metabolism by altering insulin signal transduction. This data provides a possible molecular link between low-grade systemic inflammation and insulin resistance [64]. Patients with diabetes showed high mRNA and protein expression of TNF-α in skeletal muscle and increased TNF-α levels in plasma; and it is likely that adipose tissue, which produces TNF-α, is the main source of the circulating TNF-α in chronic inflammation [65]. Because TNF-α mainly works locally, TNF-α transcription may not always be reflected in enhanced systemic levels of TNF-α [67]. In this sense, it has been suggested that chronically elevated levels of IL-6, IL-1ra, and CRP are likely to reflect local ongoing TNF-α production [68].

When findings regarding IL-6 in low-grade chronic inflammation are analyzed, results shown in the bibliography are, at least, controversial. Several studies suggest a link between IL-6 and insulin resistance. However, the evaluation of the metabolic effects of physiological concentrations of IL-6 in humans demonstrates that IL-6 enhances glucose uptake and induces fat oxidation. It has been suggested that IL-6 promotes insulin resistance due to the observation that plasma IL-6 is often elevated in patients with metabolic disease

[50]. At resting conditions, acute IL-6 administration at physiological concentrations did not impair whole-body glucose disposal, net leg-glucose uptake, or increased endogenous glucose production in resting healthy young humans [69-71]. In patients with type 2 diabetes, plasma-insulin decreased in response to IL-6 infusion, suggesting an insulin-sensitizing effect of IL-6 [71]. Carey *et al.* demonstrated that IL-6 increased the glucose infusion rate and glucose oxidation without affecting the suppression of endogenous glucose production during a hyperinsulinemic euglycemic clamp in healthy humans [47]. Infusion of recombinant human IL-6 into healthy humans to obtain physiological concentrations of IL-6 increased lipolysis in the absence of high triacylglyceride levels or changes in catecholamines, glucagon, insulin, or any adverse effects in healthy individuals [70-72] and in patients with type 2 diabetes [71]. These findings, as well as others demonstrate that IL-6 alone markedly increases both lipolysis and fat oxidation in cell cultures, that suggest IL-6 could be considered as a novel lipolytic factor. Blocking IL-6 in clinical trials with patients with rheumatoid arthritis leads to enhanced cholesterol and plasma glucose levels, indicating that functional lack of IL-6 may lead to insulin resistance and an atherogenic lipid profile rather than the opposite [73, 74]. Thus, more studies are necessary in order to clarify the relationship between high permanent IL-6 plasma levels and the incidence or development of chronic diseases.

Interestingly, tumor initiation, promotion, and progression are stimulated by systemic elevation of pro-inflammatory cytokines [53]. In addition, evidence exists to suggest that inflammation accelerates cancer cell growth [75]. The association between inflammation and cancer has been clearly illustrated by epidemiologic and clinical studies [75-77]. For instance, the risk of colorectal cancer was 10-fold greater when linked with inflammatory bowel disease, such as ulcerative colitis and Crohn's disease [78, 79]. Moreover, the control of colitis by a number of anti-inflammatory agents reduced colon cancer incidence [80, 81], and people who have taken non-steroidal anti-inflammatory drugs are at reduced risk of colon cancer [82, 83]. Direct evidence for the involvement of TNF-α in malignancy comes from the observation that mice lacking the gene for TNF-α are resistant to skin carcinogenesis [84]. TNF-α activates nuclear factor ΚB (NF-ΚB), and more recently, it has become clear that NF-ΚB signaling also has a critical role in cancer development and progression. NF-ΚB could supposedly be the link between inflammation and cancer and is a major factor controlling the ability of both pre-neoplastic and malignant cells to resist apoptosis based tumor surveillance mechanisms [85].

Chapter 4

ACUTE EFFECTS OF EXERCISE ON IMMUNE FUNCTION

Physical activity, inflammation, and immunity are tightly linked in an interesting and complex way [86]. Regular, moderate exercise reduces systemic inflammation [41]. The mediators of this beneficial effect of exercise are unclear; however, several candidate mechanisms have been identified. First, exercise increases the release of epinephrine, cortisol, growth hormone and other factors that have immuno-modulatory effects [87]. Furthermore, exercise results in decreased expression of Toll-like receptor on monocytes suggest being involved in mediating whole body inflammation [88]. In contrast to the reduction of chronic inflammation by regular, moderate exercise, prolonged, high intensity training results in increased systemic inflammation and elevated risk of infection [41]. In fact, subsequent to this type of exercise, athletes exhibit a transient exercise-induced immuno-depression [89]. The anti-inflammatory effects of exercise will be discussed later.

It is well recognized that intense exercise causes perturbations to the immune system. Long-duration or damaging exercise initiates reactions that resemble the acute-phase response to infection [41, 90]. It has been suggested that this immune response is necessary for muscular regeneration and adaptation to physical exercise [91, 92]. Although results regarding effects of exercise on immune cells functionality are controversial, emphasis the effects of exercise on the number of immunocompetent cells during the acute phase response have been well described. An increase in neurophil number (neutrophilia) is well documented after an acute bout of exercise [41, 93-96]. However, lymphocyte concentration increases during exercise but falls below basal values after intense or long duration exercises [41, 87, 93-95, 97]. Furthermore, exercise induces redistribution in lymphocyte populations [90]. The magnitude of these changes is basically related to both the intensity and duration of exercise [93].

Although moderate exercise stimulates the immune system, strenuous exercise induces a temporary immune depression in the recovery period and may explain the increased risk of infection in athletes [98]. In a few studies involving strenuous (marathons) or very extreme exercise (such as ultra-marathons), this immune depression has been associated with an increased incidence of infection in the weeks following the event [99-102]. The mechanisms underlying exercise-associated immune changes are multi-factorial and include neuroendocrinological factors such as adrenaline, noradrenaline, epinephrine, growth hormone, and cortisol [41, 98, 103]. In fact, the response to exercise includes hormonal changes which could influence immune function [41, 93]. These hormonal changes include increases in the plasma concentration of adrenaline, cortisol, and growth hormone, and are known to have immuno-modulatory effects [93].

Exercise also causes increases in the plasma concentrations of various non-hormonal substances that are known to influence leukocyte functions, including inflammatory cytokines, such as macrophage inflammatory protein-1, and IL-1□; anti-inflammatory cytokines IL-6, IL-10, and IL-1ra; and acute phase proteins, including CRP [41]. As it will be discussed later, the large increase in plasma IL-6 concentration observed during exercise can be entirely attributed to the release of this cytokine from exercising muscle [42-44]. This IL-6 release could play an essential role as the key factor in the anti-inflammatory effects of exercise.

Though an acute bout of physical activity is accompanied by responses that in many aspects are similar to those induced by infection and sepsis, there are some important differences in the cytokine response to exercise from that induced by severe infection [41, 98, 104, 105]. These differences could be essential in order to understand the possible anti-inflammatory effects of exercise. As it has been indicated previously, the initial cytokines as they appear in the circulation in relation to an acute infection consist of (named in order): TNF-α, IL-1β, IL-6, IL-1ra, sTNF-R, and IL-10. The most important, and essential, difference between exercise and sepsis with regard to cytokine responses is that the pro-inflammatory cytokines, TNF-α and IL-1β, in general do not increase with exercise.

Chapter 5

ACUTE EXERCISE AND CIRCULATING CYTOKINE LEVELS

The fact that the pro-inflammatory cytokines, TNF-α and IL-1β, in general do not increase with exercise, suggests that, as it has been indicated before; the cytokine cascade induced by exercise markedly differs from the cytokine cascade induced by infections. IL-6 is the first cytokine present in the circulation during exercise, and the appearance of IL-6 in the circulation is, by far, the most marked and its appearance precedes that of the other cytokines [104]. The level of circulating IL-6 increases in an exponential way (up to 100 fold) in response to exercise, and declines in the post-exercise period [98, 104]. The magnitude by which plasma IL-6 increases is related to exercise duration, intensity, endurance capacity and muscle mass involved in the mechanical work [32, 98, 104, 106]. However, it is not related to muscle damage because a marked increase in circulating levels of IL-6 after exercise without muscle damage has been a remarkably consistent finding [32, 98, 104, 106]. Another finding in relation to exercise is the increased circulating levels of well-known anti-inflammatory cytokines, cytokine inhibitors such as IL-1ra and sTNF-R [105, 107]. Thus, it has been shown that, in general, exercise provokes an increase primarily in IL-6, followed by an increase mainly in sTNF-R, IL-1ra, and IL-10 [32, 49, 104, 108, 109]. A small increase of CRP levels is seen the day after exhaustive exercises [98].

Regarding the response of other cytokines to exercise, changes observed are not as consistent as the ones previously indicated. Plasma concentration of IL-8 increases in response to exhaustive exercise such as running, which involves eccentric muscle contractions [110, 111]. However, concentric exercise, such as bicycle ergometry [112] or rowing [113] of moderate intensity, does not increase plasma IL-8 concentration. In a study by Nieman *et al.*, an increase in IL-8 mRNA was found in skeletal muscle biopsies from subjects having completed a three-hour treadmill run concomitant with increased plasma levels of IL-8 [111]. Similarly, IL-8 mRNA increased in response to 1 hour of exercise in a cycle-ergometer, but with no change in the plasma concentration of IL-8 [112]. Akerstom *et al.* found that IL-8 protein was clearly expressed in human skeletal muscle in response to concentric exercise [114]. The finding of a marked increase of IL-8 mRNA in muscle biopsies during and following exercise and IL-8 protein expression within skeletal muscle fibers in the recovery from exercise indicates that exercise stimulates muscle cells to produce IL-8; which, in addition, exerts its effects locally [114]. These results are in accordance with the finding that muscle cells *in vitro* have the capacity to express IL-8, both at the mRNA and protein levels [115]. In fact, it has been proposed that IL-8 should be classified as a myokine [114].

The physiological function of IL-8 within the muscle is still unknown. It is well know that IL-8 attracts primarily neutrophils and, in addition, IL-8 acts as an angiogenic factor [116]. The main part of the systemic increase in IL-8 as seen during exercise with an eccentric component is most likely because of an inflammatory response. In fact, not all the studies found increases in plasma IL-8 concentration during or after concentric exercise [111-114]. However, when the arterio-venous concentration difference across a concentrically exercising limb was measured, a small and transient net release of IL-8, which does not result in an increase in the systemic IL-8 plasma concentration has been detected [114]. The high local IL-8 expression taking place in working muscle with only a small and transient release could indicate that muscle-derived IL-8 acts locally and exerts its effect in an endocrine or paracrine fashion. Taking into account these results, it was suggested that a plausible function of the muscle-derived IL-8 would be chemo attraction of neutrophils and macrophages when, in fact, in concentric exercise there is little or no accumulation of neutrophils or macrophages in skeletal muscle.

Levels of IL-15 mRNA were found to be higher in human skeletal muscles dominated by type-2 muscle fibers than in muscles dominated by type-1 muscle fibers, and that IL-15 mRNA content increased 24 hours following a bout of resistance exercise [117]. The increase in IL-15 mRNA levels was not accompanied by an increase in muscular IL-15 protein expression, neither was plasma IL-15 protein increased after a bout of resistance exercise. This was in contrast to Riechman *et al.* [118] that demonstrated a small, but significant increase in plasma IL-15 protein following resistance exercise. They found an increase in plasma IL-15 immediately after the end of a resistance exercise bout.

A third study in humans did not find any change in IL-15 mRNA level in muscle biopsies obtained immediately after exercise. However, the strength training in this study influenced *vastus lateralis* to only a minor degree [119], possibly explaining the discrepancy. IL-15 has anabolic effects on muscle cell culture and decreases the muscle degradation rate in a cachexia model, suggesting that IL-15 might be of importance in muscle growth [120]. Furthermore, IL-15 has been suggested to play a role in muscle-adipose tissue interaction [121]. Thus, it is not known if IL-15 is an essential component in exercise-induced immuno-regulation. However, the findings that IL-15 is constitutively expressed by skeletal muscle and regulated by strength training, together with the finding that IL-15 has anabolic effects and seems to play a role in reducing adipose tissue mass. This could indicate that IL-15 may play a role in muscle-fat cross talk [117], possibly reducing inflammation by means of a decrease in circulating lipids.

Several studies have examined the effects of both acute and chronic exercise on serum CRP levels. Regarding changes induced by an acute bout of exercise, studies in marathon runners have found that strenuous acute exercise produces large transient increases in CRP [122]. CRP highest levels are usually found 24 hours after exercise. The finding of increased circulating CRP levels after exercise is consistent across most studies and is probably due to the exercise-induced release of IL-6 and other pro-inflammatory cytokines from skeletal muscle that regulate CRP production in the liver [29].

Chapter 6

ANTI-INFLAMMATORY RESPONSE INDUCED BY ACUTE EXERCISE: ROLE OF IL-6

Extensive research has shown that during and immediately after exercise, there is a significant increase in plasma IL-6, where in the hours following exercise, is accompanied by an increase in the anti-inflammatory cytokines IL-10 [105, 123] and IL-1ra [32, 49, 104, 108, 109]. Furthermore, acute prolonged exercise has been shown to increase the expression of the oxidant-responsive anti-inflammatory gene HO-1 in lymphocytes [124, 125]. During acute exercise, working muscles release a number of cytokines into the circulation, including IL-6 that may modulate systemic low-level inflammation [107]. The exercise-induced increase in IL-6 stimulates the appearance of other anti-inflammatory cytokines, including IL-1ra, sTNFR, and IL-10; whereas circulating levels of pro-inflammatory cytokines, such as TNF-α and IL-1, are generally not increased by acute exercise [29].

As it has been described, the increase of IL-6 is independent on concomitant muscle damage and the magnitude by which plasma IL-6 increases is related to exercise duration, intensity, the muscle mass involved in the mechanical work, and the endurance capacity. Even moderate exercise has major effects on muscle-derived IL-6 [126, 127]. The IL-6 mRNA is up-regulated in contracting skeletal muscle [42, 111, 128-132] and the transcriptional rate of the IL-6 gene is markedly enhanced by exercise, especially when muscle glycogen levels are low [133]. It has also been demonstrated that the IL-6 protein is expressed after exercise in muscle fibers [134], and that IL-6 is released from skeletal muscle during exercise [44]. Exercise was also found to increase IL-6 receptor production in human skeletal muscle, suggest a possible post-exercise sensitizing mechanism to IL-6 [48]. It has been suggested that IL-6 acts as an autocrine factor up-regulating its mRNA levels, thereby supporting its function as an exercise activated factor in skeletal muscle cells [45]. Unlike IL-6 signaling in macrophages, intramuscular IL-6 expression is regulated by a network of signaling events that among other pathways are likely to involve the production of nitric oxide (NO) [135] and Ca^{2+} [136] following muscle contraction and p38 MAPK pathways regarding reduction of the glycogen content [137].

In spite of IL-6 classified as a pro-inflammatory cytokine, recent data suggest that IL-6 and IL-6-regulated acute phase proteins are anti-inflammatory and immune-suppressive, and may negatively regulate the acute phase response [138]. It has been shown that the exercise induced increase in plasma IL-6 is followed by increased circulating levels of well-known anti-inflammatory cytokines, such as IL-1ra and IL-10 [107]. The cytokine response to exercise has been replicated by using an infusion of IL-6 to healthy donors that also increase the systemic levels of cortisol [139].

Some studies have found results pointing to inhibitory effects of IL-6 on TNF-α and IL-1β production. It has been shown that IL-6 inhibits lipopolysaccharide (LPS)-induced TNF-α production both in cultured human monocytes and in the human monocytic line U937 [140], indicating that circulating IL-6 is involved in the regulation of TNF-α levels. Furthermore, Starkie et al. showed that IL-6 stimulates the release of soluble TNF-α receptors, but not IL-1β and TNF-α [141]. They also suggest that IL-6 was the primary inducer of the hepatocyte-derived acute-phase proteins, many of which have anti-inflammatory properties. Interestingly, both exercise and IL-6 infusion suppress TNF-α production in humans [141]. Both, in vitro [142] and animal [143, 144] studies have also suggested the role of IL-6 inhibiting TNF-α production.

The appearance of IL-10 and IL-1ra in the circulation after exercise contributes to the anti-inflammatory effects of exercise [29]. The anti-inflammatory properties of IL-10 derived from the ability to inhibit the production of the pro-inflammatory cytokines IL-1α, IL-1β, and TNF-α; as well as the production of several pro-inflammatory chemokynes, especially in monocytes and neutrophils [36, 37, 145]. Interestingly, it has been shown that while IL-10 inhibits cytokine synthesis in mononuclear cells acting mainly at the level of cytokine gene transcription [37], the IL-8 production is prevented by affecting both gene transcription and mRNA stability [36]. All these compounds are essential in the activation of most of the immune cells and their recruitment to the sites of inflammation. Then, it can be suggested that the exercise induced increases in IL-10 and limits the inflammatory response by preventing the appearance of several pro-inflammatory cytokines and chemokynes. The IL-1ra appearance in circulation after exercise could contribute to the anti-inflammatory effects of exercise because, as it has been indicated previously, the role of IL-1ra is to inhibit signaling transduction through the IL-1 receptor complex, preventing the production of the pro-inflammatory cytokines IL-1α, IL-1β [39]. CRP has been also described as an anti-inflammatory compound because of its role in both the induction of anti-inflammatory cytokines and in the suppression of the synthesis of pro-inflammatory cytokines [146]. As well as IL-10 and IL-1ra, CRP has been suggested to increase after exercise, at least in part, due to IL-6 induction [29].

Taking into account these results, we can conclude that exercise induces, via IL-6, an anti-inflammatory environment by inducing the production of IL-1ra and IL-10, and the inhibition of the TNF-α production. However, exercise is likely to suppress TNF-α also via IL-6-independent pathways, as demonstrated by the finding of a modest decrease of TNF-α following exercise in IL-6 KO mice [147]. As discussed in Chapter 5, exercise induces high levels of epinephrine, and epinephrine infusion has been shown to prevent the appearance of TNF-α in response to endotoxin *in vivo* [148]. As epinephrine infusion induces only a small increase in IL-6 [149], the mechanism whereby epinephrine inhibits TNF-α production is not clear. However, authors of these works suggest that epinephrine and IL-6 inhibit the endotoxin-induced appearance of TNF-α via independent mechanisms. Interestingly, it has recently been demonstrated that epinephrine infusion also increased IL-10 release [148], indicating a possible contribution of epinephrine to the anti-inflammatory environment after exercise.

In a very interesting and innovative study, the existence of a true anti-inflammatory response to exercise, as well as the role of IL-6, was analyzed in a model of "low-grade inflammation" based on the administration of a low dose of *Escherichia coli* endotoxin to healthy volunteers [141]. To test the hypotheses that IL-6 as well as physical exercise inhibits TNF-α production, eight healthy males participated in three experiments where they rested or performed bicycling for three hours or were infused with recombinant IL-6 (rhIL-6) for three hours while they rested. After 2.5 hours, the volunteers received a bolus of *E. Coli* lipopolysaccharide endotoxin intravenously to induce low grade inflammation. In the control study, plasma TNF-α increased significantly in response to endotoxin. In contrast, in subjects with high levels of IL-6, induced by the exercise or by the rhIL-6 infusion, the endotoxin-induced increase in TNF-α was completely abolished. Thus, this study demonstrated that physical exercise inhibits the production of TNF-α elicited by low-grade endotoxemia in humans and suggested that exercise-induced IL-6 production may contribute to mediate the effect of exercise on endotoxin-induced TNF-α production. Finally, authors of the study suggest that IL-6 plays an essential role mediating the anti-inflammatory effects of exercise [141].

INFLUENCE OF EXERCISE INTENSITY AND DURATION

Some studies utilizing moderate-intensity exercise have shown that exercise elicits changes in certain inflammatory markers, and others have found no effect [150-152]. Nieman *et al.* [150] demonstrated a modest increase in total leukocyte count and plasma IL-6 concentration one hour following a 30-min treadmill walk at 60-65% VO_2max in young women who were accustomed to regular walking. It is not clear whether differences in subject characteristics (sex, age, or fitness) or exercise intensity (50% vs. 60-65% VO_2max) explain this apparent discrepancy. Only a few studies have investigated the effect of moderate-intensity exercise on plasma concentrations of the anti-inflammatory cytokine IL-10. As an example, the systemic concentration of IL-10 in young well-trained male runners did not change following one hour of running at 60% VO_2max [153]. However, as it has been indicated before, even moderate exercise induces increases in plasma IL-6 [126, 127].

No effect on the expression of the anti-inflammatory protein HO-1 in lymphocytes or in lymphocyte adhesion to cultured endothelial cells was found after a protocol of moderate exercise [154]. Lymphocyte HO-1 expression is up-regulated in response to prolonged demanding exercise [124, 125], but eccentric contractions and a short exhaustive run have been shown to have no effect on HO-1 protein expression in leukocytes [1]. *In vitro* adhesion assays have been used to demonstrate a reduction in lymphocyte adhesion to human umbilical venous endothelial cells in middle-age healthy individuals following a short cycle ergometer exercise at 75% VO_2max, which was accompanied by a significant increase in serum IL-6 concentrations immediately after finishing exercise [152]. It seems that exercise intensity and duration are both important in determining the inflammatory response to exercise, with intensity being particularly important. Markovitch *et al.* did not observe an inflammatory response following a 30-min walking protocol at 50% VO_2max [154]. Other studies show that exercise of a shorter or similar duration can elicit an inflammatory response, but only if the intensity is higher [155, 156]. Similarly, low-intensity protocols that are very prolonged in duration (1-legged dynamic knee extensor exercise for five hours at 40% VO_2max) also induce an inflammatory response [44]. In their work, Markovitch *et al.* pointed that studies using more intense exercise protocols tend to use younger and fitter individuals, and this means that not only is there a difference in terms of relative work rate (e.g., 50% VO_2max vs. 60% VO_2max), but there will be an even more pronounced difference in absolute work rate because of an age-related decline in capacity (e.g., in absolute running speeds or METs). The conclusion of this interesting work is that a single bout of moderate-intensity exercise of a duration that would meet public health recommendations in middle-aged men was insufficient to induce a pro- or anti-inflammatory response [154]. Taking this and other results into account, it is suggested that some kind of intensity or duration threshold must be achieved to elicit an acute change in measures such as IL-6 and IL-10 [154].

Chapter 7

ANTI-INFLAMMATORY EFFECTS OF CHRONIC MODERATE EXERCISE

As it has been indicated previously, clinically there is general evidence supporting a beneficial effect of continuous moderate physical activity in patients with chronic diseases or metabolic disorders [22]. However, it would be interesting to clarify to what extend how regular moderate exercise benefits patients with chronic diseases and how it can be attributed to anti-inflammatory exercise effects. Studies examining the effects of chronic exercise on cytokine production and circulating cytokine levels present contradictory results [49] and, in general, do not clarify the possible mechanisms involved.

Several chronic diseases and metabolism related disorders involve high TNF-α levels. TNF-α reduces muscle strength by affecting myocite differentiation and inducing cachexia [157]. Both COPD and rheumatoid arthritis are characterized by high circulating TNF-α levels and muscle strength lost [56, 57]. It has been suggested that exercise training could prevent muscle strength lost in these patients because of the exercise induced release of IL-6 [22]. Furthermore, the IL-6 inhibition of TNF-α production; and, in general, the IL-6 induced anti-inflammatory environment [106] could be the responsible for the positive effects of exercise in patients with chronic diseases characterized by high levels of inflammatory cytokines. In fact, cross-sectional studies show that increasing levels of physical activity and/or fitness are generally associated with modest decreases in circulating levels of CRP, TNF-α, and IL-6, and increased levels of IL-10 [158, 159]. In agreement with these results, Smith *et al.* [160] observed a significant reduction in the production of the pro-inflammatory cytokines IFN-γ, TNF-α, and IL-1β, and a significant increase in the production of the anti-inflammatory cytokines TGF-β (transforming growth factor-β), IL-4 and IL-10, by cultured mononuclear cells from persons at risk of developing ischemic heart disease after six months of programmed physical activity when compared with production before exercise. Subjects in this study followed an individualized, supervised exercise program, with a mean of 2.5 hours of exercise per week. Smith et al. also observed a possible dose-response relationship between some of the changes observed and the time subjects spent performing some types of exercise [160]. However, in order to discuss this last result, it should be noted that only 43 subjects completed the study. Recently, Sanders et al. evaluated the associations between physical activity and inflammatory markers (CRP and IL-1β) in patients with periodontitis as well as in healthy subjects [161]. They found that increased physical activity was associated with lower levels of CRP in subjects with periodontitis; however, they indicated that this association was not apparent in healthy subjects [161]. Some studies demonstrate reduced circulating levels of TNF-α, IL-6, IFN-γ and other markers of systemic inflammation after exercise training programs, but these did not indicate any effect [159]. It has been suggested that these discrepancies may be due to a number of factors, including differences in subject characteristics, the type and intensity of the exercise intervention, the timing of the blood samples taken and inherent variability in the assays used to measure many of these cytokines [49]. However, it has been also indicated that the preponderance of evidence suggests that both acute and chronic exercise is associated with modest improvements in markers of systemic low-grade inflammation [49]. In this sense, chronic exercise has been hypothesized to reduce circulating levels of CRP and other inflammatory markers. In fact, most of the studies focused on the effects of continuous moderate exercise on inflammation have used plasma CRP as inflammatory marker. A decrease in plasma CRP levels is considered an indicator of decreased systemic inflammation. Cross-sectional studies demonstrate an association between physical inactivity and low-grade systemic inflammation in healthy subjects [160, 162-168], in elderly people [169], and in patients with intermittent claudication [170]. These correlational data do not, however, provide any information with regard to a possible causal relationship. However, the finding in longitudinal studies that regular training induces a reduction in CRP level suggests that physical activity may suppress systemic low grade inflammation [162, 163, 171, 172].

Data from prospective studies examining the effect of exercise training on CRP levels have been inconclusive. Smith et al. found a 35% decrease in serum levels of CRP after a 6-month exercise program [160]. This data suggested that the decrease observed was as a result of changes in blood mononuclear cells function observed after the six month of exercise (as it has been previously discussed) [160]. In a meta-analysis of randomized controlled clinical trials published in 2006, Kelley *et al.* concluded that aerobic exercise training does not reduce basal CRP levels [173]. This meta-analysis included data from 323 male and female subjects in five independent trials in which subjects were randomized to either a control group or an aerobic exercise intervention (171 exercise and 152 control) lasting at least 4 weeks. Results showed a non-significant reduction of about 3% in CRP levels in the exercise groups after exercise training. Kohut *et al.* [174] randomly assigned adults (64 years old) to either an aerobic exercise program or a flexibility/strength exercise treatment for 10 months. They found that the aerobic exercise program significantly reduced serum CRP by 10-15% [174]. Furthermore, the aerobic program resulted in significant reductions when compared with the decrease observed after the flexibility/strength exercise. Both, IL-6 and IL-18 in this study followed the same pattern of change as CRP. After reviewing data from several longitudinal studies, Plaisance and Grandjean [158] suggested that long-term exercise training significantly reduces plasma CRP levels. They suggested that this positive effect could be independent of baseline CRP levels, body composition and weight loss [158], which could be some of the confounding factors in these studies regarding the mechanisms for the positive effects of exercise. It has been suggested that the clinical significance of these improvements is uncertain because they may not reflect changes occurring at the tissue level. But, on the other hand, it has been also suggested that a change in the tissue concentration of certain chemokynes, which work at local level, could not be reflected in the circulating levels but could produce either positive or negative effects [68].

In addition to these studies, others have demonstrated interesting and healthy relations between different programs of regular physical activity or training programs and inflammatory markers (CRP and others). In this sense both epidemiological and clinical data evidenced positive effects of physical activity [165, 167, 175-177]. In a cohort of 5,888 men and women over 65 years of age, higher levels of self-reported physical activity were associated with lower serum concentrations of several markers of inflammation, including CRP and fibrinogen, as well as lower white blood cell counts, after adjusting for age, sex, race, presence of cardiovascular disease, smoking, BMI, diabetes, and hypertension [165]. This data suggests that increased exercise is associated with reduced inflammation [165]. Cross-sectional studies consistently demonstrate an inverse relationship between plasma CRP and both physical activity level and cardio-respiratory fitness [178]. These associations remain after controlling for potential confounders in some studies [175], although others suggest they may be influenced by factors, such as gender, body composition and the type of physical activity among others .

As it has been suggested earlier, no relationship between physical activity levels and CRP is found in some studies after adjusting for BMI (body mass index) and other risk factors [181, 182]. In this sense, Arsenault et al. [183] recently showed that after adjusting for visceral adipose tissue, fitness was not associated with variation in inflammatory markers. This study suggested that the previously reported association between poor fitness and low-grade inflammation may be largely attributable to increased visceral adipose tissue accumulation and its associated state of insulin resistance, conditions frequently observed in subjects with poor cardio-respiratory fitness [183]. As it has been emphasized previously, weight loss could be an important confounding factor in these studies. In fact, it has been consistently reported that weight loss induces a decrease in CRP levels [184]. Most exercise training interventions have shown modest or no effects on CRP after statistically correcting for weight loss, but few studies have assessed the effect of exercise on CRP in the absence of weight loss [184]. In the same way, Hammet et al. [188] studied the effects of exercise training on five inflammatory markers associated with cardiovascular risk (including fibrinogen and CRP) in 152 healthy female smokers. The exercise group took part in three 45-minute supervised exercise sessions per week using different ergometers (cycle, treadmill and rowing). They found that the exercise training improved cardio-respiratory fitness but had no consistent effect on inflammatory marker levels. Because they found that baseline associations between physical fitness and inflammatory markers were largely explained by differences in body fat, they suggested that associations between greater physical fitness and lower inflammatory markers may be explained by long-term regular exercise reducing body and visceral fat [188], which is the main reason some authors suggest decreased inflammation after an exercise training program.

Several studies have shown a significant inverse relationship between physical fitness and plasma IL-6 [185], whereas plasma IL-10, an anti-inflammatory cytokine, is positively related to fitness [186]. As in CRP, and in spite of IL-6 has been recognized an anti-inflammatory cytokine, continuous increased IL-6 levels are considered as a marker of low-grade systemic inflammation. Thus, a decrease in basal IL-6 circulating levels would be a healthy achievement. In an analysis of 880 participants aged between 70 and 79 years, Taaffe et al. showed found that both serum IL-6 and CRP concentrations were inversely associated with the hours per year undertaking moderate and strenuous physical activity; and, also, with aerobic fitness as measured by the distance covered in six minutes of fast walking [167]. Survival seven years later was associated with lower baseline IL-6 concentrations and also greater baseline six-minute walking distances [167]. The effects of physical activity on inflammatory cytokine activity persist even when obesity is considered. It is well known that obesity is associated with increased production of pro-inflammatory cytokines [65, 67]. Hotamisligil *et al.* [65] showed first in animal models that TNF-α protein was elevated locally and systemically in obese animal models, indicating a role for TNF-α in obesity. In an analysis of 27,158 apparently healthy adult women (mean age 54.7 years) from the Women's Health Study, which found significant associations between BMI and several inflammatory and lipid markers, including serum concentrations of CRP, fibrinogen, soluble intracellular adhesion molecule-1 (sICAM-1), total cholesterol, and low-density lipoprotein [177]. As expected, high density lipoprotein cholesterol (HDL-C) concentrations decreased with increasing BMI [177]. However, physical activity was associated with small but significant reductions in the serum concentrations of these biomarkers compared with inactive individuals, (except HDL-C, which increased slightly), independent of BMI [177]. This beneficial effect was strongest on inflammatory markers, such as CRP and fibrinogen, as compared to lipid biomarkers [177]. In a study involving high-intensity training, Mattusch *et al.* examined the effects of a nine-month increased training program in preparation for a marathon [163]. CRP was reduced about 31% in highly trained runners after the nine months of increased training but did not change significantly in non-training control subjects. Although the reduction in CRP in the training group in this study was statistically significant, authors indicated that the physiological relevance of such a small absolute change in CRP levels is unknown [163]. Furthermore, it was suggested that because the subjects in the 'training' group were already highly fit runners, the significance of these findings to the general population is also uncertain [49]. In a cohort of 3,075 elderly men and women (aged 70-79) from the Health, Aging and Body Composition Study, higher levels of exercise were associated with lower concentrations of CRP, IL-6, and TNF-α in subjects not taking antioxidant supplements [187]. However, in one of the longest randomized controlled trial Rauramaa *et al.* did not find any significant effect of low to moderate intensity training on plasma CRP levels [180]. After six years of exercise training they found a non-significant decrease in plasma CRP levels in the exercise group in spite of the increase observed in the ventilatory aerobic threshold [180].

As indicated previously, the type of physical activity could be one of the confounding factors when results of these studies are analyzed. Some studies have examined and compared the relationship between different types of exercise and CRP levels. King *et al.* (in the Third National Health and Nutrition Examination

Survey) [166], found that different aerobic exercises (e.g., jogging, swimming, cycling, aerobic dancing) were associated with lower CRP levels. However, after controlling for possible confounding factors such as age, race, sex and BMI, only regular participants in jogging and aerobic dancing showed still significant lower CRP levels [166]. Dufaux *et al.* [179] concluded that exercise training induces a decrease in CRP circulating levels in both male and female swimmers when compared to controls. However, they find non-significant lower levels in rowers, cyclists, and football players [179]. Kohut *et al.* [174] found that both, an aerobic and a flexibility/strength exercise programs induced significant decreases in TNF-α plasma levels after ten months of exercise training. Sloan *et al.* [189] examined the anti-inflammatory effects of exercise by measuring monocyte TNF-α production after a 12-week aerobic training program. Blood was taken before and after a moderate or high intensity training schedule and, then, it was stimulated *ex vivo* by addition of lipopolysaccharide. The authors found that exercise training induced a decrease in TNF-α production only in the high intensity training group. However, authors of this study did not measure any other inflammatory or anti-inflammatory marker or possible mediators in the mechanism involved.

Finally, it is also possible that gender influences effects of exercise on inflammatory markers. Several studies have found differences between the effects of training on CRP levels in males and females [179, 190, 191]. Some of these observational studies indicate that chronic physical activity reduces CRP levels more in males than females [179, 190, 191]. However, Arsenault *et al.* [183] reported that fitness did not correlate with any of the individual inflammatory markers in men, whereas it was negatively associated with CRP and IL-6 in women. They indicate that more studies are necessary to explain the basis of gender differences.

MECHANISMS INVOLVED IN THE ANTI-INFLAMMATORY EFFECT OF MODERATE EXERCISE

It has been suggested that regular physical activity is anti-inflammatory partly because of the changes induced by each individual bout of exercise [29, 138]. In this sense, with regular exercise, the anti-inflammatory effects of an acute bout of exercise will protect against chronic systemic low-grade inflammation, but such a link between the acute effects of exercise and the long-term benefits has not yet been proven. Vigorous exercise elevates serum IL-6 concentration, which may be anti-inflammatory through the increased production of IL-1ra and IL-10 [29].

Furthermore, vigorous exercise increases the lymphocyte expression of the anti-inflammatory enzyme HO-1 [124, 125]. However, several studies did not find any anti-inflammatory response after an acute bout of moderate-intensity exercise protocols. For example, Markovitch *et al.* did not find any change in CRP, IL-6, IL-10, lymphocyte HO-1, or lymphocyte adhesion levels over a 7-day period in response to a single bout of moderate-intensity exercise [154].

The Markovitch *et al.* study [154] indicated that, as it had been suggested previously, it was possible that some of the benefits derived from such activity are largely related to acute changes induced by the last bout of activity. For example, the regular up-regulation of anti-inflammatory molecules such as HO-1 may contribute to an overall down-regulation of pro-atherogenic inflammatory pathways in the same way that acute regular changes in lipid metabolism may play a role in the long-term benefits of regular exercise [192]. This hypothesis seems to be adequate when demanding exercise is performed because, as it has discussed previously, an anti-inflammatory environment is generated after an acute bout of demanding exercise. However, there is less evidence that this is relevant to moderate-intensity physical activity as described in most physical activity recommendations. Taking into account their results, Markovitch *et al.* concluded that even though regular moderate-intensity exercise appears to be associated with reduced markers of inflammation in cross-sectional comparisons [185, 193, 194], this does not appear to be explained by acute inflammatory changes induced by each exercise bout because they did not find any change after an acute bout of moderate exercise. Authors of this study suggested that other mechanisms inducing the anti-inflammatory effect of long-term, moderate-intensity exercise should be considered and examined in future studies. They also suggested that it seems that other changes associated with regular moderate-intensity exercise ultimately explain the anti-inflammatory effect. For example, a reduction in body mass following a controlled physical activity program [195] or fat mass through dietary intervention [196] can be anti-inflammatory and reduce chronic inflammation. Furthermore, positive changes in lipid and glycemic profiles could also explain the anti-inflammatory effect of regular moderate-intensity exercise [197]. In fact, there is considerable evidence that independently of weight loss, physical activity has beneficial effects on patients with dyslipidemia, improving the blood lipid profile [22]. In training studies, an increase in high-density lipoprotein (HDL) and a decrease in low-density lipoprotein (LDL) are consistent findings [22]. The decrease in LDL could be an essential event in the anti-inflammatory effects of exercise in the prevention of atherosclerosis. High LDL levels are an important cardiovascular risk factor which can initiate the development of atherosclerosis even in the absence of other risk factors [49]. When circulating levels are elevated, LDL can accumulate in the sub-endothelial space, where it becomes oxidized [49]. The oxidative modification of LDL (ox-LDL) promotes an inflammatory response, recruitment of macrophages and the development of atherosclerotic lesions. The inflammation initiated by ox-LDL is mediated by the local production of pro-inflammatory cytokines in the artery wall [49]. Thus, if exercise reduces LDL circulating levels, it also could reduce LDL oxidation, ox-LDL induced inflammatory response and, as a consequence, atherosclerosis development.

CONCLUSION

There is important evidence regarding the positive effects of regular exercise in patients with chronic diseases but also in the prevention of the diseases. Low grade systemic inflammation has been found to be involved in several chronic diseases which suppose the largest cause of death in the world. Recent findings have demonstrated that an acute bout of physical activity induces an anti-inflammatory response, where muscles play an essential role via IL-6 production. Furthermore, there is substantial evidence regarding the anti-inflammatory effects of continuous moderate-intensity physical activity. However, mechanisms underlying these positive effects remain unclear and need to be examined further.

REFERENCES

[1] Fehrenbach, E; Niess, AM; Passek, F; Sorichter, S; Schwirtz, A; Berg, A; Dickhuth, HH; Northoff, H. Influence of different types of exercise on the expression of haem oxygenase-1 in leukocytes. *J Sports Sci*, 2003, 21, 383-9.

[2] Department of Health and Human Services, CfDCaP, National Center for Chronic Disease Prevention and Health Promotion. Physical Activity and Health: A Report of the Surgeon General. Atlanta: GA: DHHS, 1996.

[3] Hu, G; Tuomilehto, J; Silventoinen, K; Barengo, NC; Peltonen, M; Jousilahti, P. The effects of physical activity and body mass index on cardiovascular, cancer and all-cause mortality among 47212 middle-aged Finnish men and women. *Int J Obes (Lond)*, 2005, 29, 894-902.

[4] Lees, SJ; Booth, FW. Physical inactivity is a disease. *World Rev Nutr Diet*, 2005, 95, 73-9.

[5] Thompson, PD; Buchner, D; Pina, IL; Balady, GJ; Williams, MA; Marcus, BH; Berra, K; Blair, SN; Costa, F; Franklin, B; Fletcher, GF; Gordon, NF; Pate, RR; Rodriguez, BL; Yancey, AK; Wenger, NK. Exercise and physical activity in the prevention and treatment of atherosclerotic cardiovascular disease: a statement from the Council on Clinical Cardiology (Subcommittee on Exercise, Rehabilitation, and Prevention) and the Council on Nutrition, Physical Activity, and Metabolism (Subcommittee on Physical Activity). *Circulation*, 2003, 107, 3109-16.

[6] Myers, J; Kaykha, A; George, S; Abella, J; Zaheer, N; Lear, S; Yamazaki, T; Froelicher, V. Fitness versus physical activity patterns in predicting mortality in men. *Am J Med*, 2004, 117, 912-8.

[7] Church, TS; Cheng, YJ; Earnest, CP; Barlow, CE; Gibbons, LW; Priest, EL; Blair, SN. Exercise capacity and body composition as predictors of mortality among men with diabetes. *Diabetes Care*, 2004, 27, 83-8.

[8]   Farrell, SW; Braun, L; Barlow, CE; Cheng, YJ; Blair, SN. The relation of body mass index, cardiorespiratory fitness, and all-cause mortality in women. *Obes Res*, 2002, 10, 417-23.

[9]   Sandvik, L; Erikssen, J; Thaulow, E; Erikssen, G; Mundal, R; Rodahl, K. Physical fitness as a predictor of mortality among healthy, middle-aged Norwegian men. *N Engl J Med*, 1993, 328, 533-7.

[10]   Stevens, J; Cai, J; Evenson, KR; Thomas, R. Fitness and fatness as predictors of mortality from all causes and from cardiovascular disease in men and women in the lipid research clinics study. *Am J Epidemiol*, 2002, 156, 832-41.

[11]   Stevens, J; Evenson, KR; Thomas, O; Cai, J; Thomas, R. Associations of fitness and fatness with mortality in Russian and American men in the lipids research clinics study. *Int J Obes Relat Metab Disord*, 2004, 28, 1463-70.

[12]   Crespo, CJ; Palmieri, MR; Perdomo, RP; McGee, DL; Smit, E; Sempos, CT; Lee, IM; Sorlie, PD. The relationship of physical activity and body weight with all-cause mortality: results from the Puerto Rico Heart Health Program. *Ann Epidemiol*, 2002, 12, 543-52.

[13]   Andersen, LB; Schnohr, P; Schroll, M; Hein, HO. All-cause mortality associated with physical activity during leisure time, work, sports, and cycling to work. *Arch Intern Med*, 2000, 160, 1621-8.

[14]   Batty, GD; Shipley, MJ; Marmot, M; Smith, GD. Physical activity and cause-specific mortality in men: further evidence from the Whitehall study. *Eur J Epidemiol*, 2001, 17, 863-9.

[15]   Batty, GD; Shipley, MJ; Marmot, M; Smith, GD. Physical activity and cause-specific mortality in men with Type 2 diabetes/impaired glucose tolerance: evidence from the Whitehall study. *Diabet Med*, 2002, 19, 580-8.

[16]   Hu, FB; Willett, WC; Li, T; Stampfer, MJ; Colditz, GA; Manson, JE. Adiposity as compared with physical activity in predicting mortality among women. *N Engl J Med*, 2004, 351, 2694-703.

[17]   Arraiz, GA; Wigle, DT; Mao, Y. Risk assessment of physical activity and physical fitness in the Canada Health Survey mortality follow-up study. *J Clin Epidemiol*, 1992, 45, 419-28.

[18]   Gregg, EW; Cauley, JA; Stone, K; Thompson, TJ; Bauer, DC; Cummings, SR; Ensrud, KE. Relationship of changes in physical activity and mortality among older women. *Jama*, 2003, 289, 2379-86.

[19]   Sundquist, K; Qvist, J; Sundquist, J; Johansson, SE. Frequent and occasional physical activity in the elderly: a 12-year follow-up study of mortality. *Am J Prev Med*, 2004, 27, 22-7.

[20] Haapanen-Niemi, N; Miilunpalo, S; Pasanen, M; Vuori, I; Oja, P; Malmberg, J. Body mass index, physical inactivity and low level of physical fitness as determinants of all-cause and cardiovascular disease mortality--16 y follow-up of middle-aged and elderly men and women. *Int J Obes Relat Metab Disord*, 2000, 24, 1465-74.

[21] Murray, CJ; Lopez, AD. Global mortality, disability, and the contribution of risk factors: Global Burden of Disease Study. *Lancet*, 1997, 349, 1436-42.

[22] Pedersen, BK; Saltin, B. Evidence for prescribing exercise as therapy in chronic disease. *Scand J Med Sci Sports*, 2006, 16 Suppl 1, 3-63.

[23] Flynn, KE; Pina, IL; Whellan, DJ; Lin, L; Blumenthal, JA; Ellis, SJ; Fine, LJ; Howlett, JG; Keteyian, SJ; Kitzman, DW; Kraus, WE; Miller, NH; Schulman, KA; Spertus, JA; O'Connor, CM; Weinfurt, KP. Effects of exercise training on health status in patients with chronic heart failure: HF-ACTION randomized controlled trial. *Jama*, 2009, 301, 1451-9.

[24] O'Connor, CM; Whellan, DJ; Lee, KL; Keteyian, SJ; Cooper, LS; Ellis, SJ; Leifer, ES; Kraus, WE; Kitzman, DW; Blumenthal, JA; Rendall, DS; Miller, NH; Fleg, JL; Schulman, KA; McKelvie, RS; Zannad, F; Pina, IL. Efficacy and safety of exercise training in patients with chronic heart failure: HF-ACTION randomized controlled trial. *Jama*, 2009, 301, 1439-50.

[25] Libby, P. Inflammation in atherosclerosis. *Nature*, 2002, 420, 868-74.

[26] Dandona, P; Aljada, A; Bandyopadhyay, A. Inflammation: the link between insulin resistance, obesity and diabetes. *Trends Immunol*, 2004, 25, 4-7.

[27] Ross, R. Atherosclerosis--an inflammatory disease. *N Engl J Med*, 1999, 340, 115-26.

[28] Festa, A; D'Agostino, R, Jr.; Tracy, RP; Haffner, SM. Elevated levels of acute-phase proteins and plasminogen activator inhibitor-1 predict the development of type 2 diabetes: the insulin resistance atherosclerosis study. *Diabetes*, 2002, 51, 1131-7.

[29] Petersen, AM; Pedersen, BK. The anti-inflammatory effect of exercise. *J Appl Physiol*, 2005, 98, 1154-62.

[30] Pedersen, BK; Febbraio, M. Muscle-derived interleukin-6--a possible link between skeletal muscle, adipose tissue, liver, and brain. *Brain Behav Immun*, 2005, 19, 371-6.

[31] Pedersen, BK; Steensberg, A; Fischer, C; Keller, C; Keller, P; Plomgaard, P; Wolsk-Petersen, E; Febbraio, M. The metabolic role of IL-6 produced during exercise: is IL-6 an exercise factor? *Proc Nutr Soc*, 2004, 63, 263-7.

[32] Pedersen, BK; Steensberg, A; Fischer, C; Keller, C; Keller, P; Plomgaard, P; Febbraio, M; Saltin, B. Searching for the exercise factor: is IL-6 a candidate? *J Muscle Res Cell Motil*, 2003, 24, 113-9.

[33] Akira, S; Kishimoto, T. IL-6 and NF-IL6 in acute-phase response and viral infection. *Immunol Rev*, 1992, 127, 25-50.

[34] Akira, S; Taga, T; Kishimoto, T. Interleukin-6 in biology and medicine. *Adv Immunol*, 1993, 54, 1-78.

[35] Dinarello, CA. Interleukin-1 and interleukin-1 antagonism. *Blood*, 1991, 77, 1627-52.

[36] Wang, P; Wu, P; Anthes, JC; Siegel, MI; Egan, RW; Billah, MM. Interleukin-10 inhibits interleukin-8 production in human neutrophils. *Blood*, 1994, 83, 2678-83.

[37] Wang, P; Wu, P; Siegel, MI; Egan, RW; Billah, MM. IL-10 inhibits transcription of cytokine genes in human peripheral blood mononuclear cells. *J Immunol*, 1994, 153, 811-6.

[38] Bogdan, C; Paik, J; Vodovotz, Y; Nathan, C. Contrasting mechanisms for suppression of macrophage cytokine release by transforming growth factor-beta and interleukin-10. *J Biol Chem*, 1992, 267, 23301-8.

[39] Dinarello, CA. The role of the interleukin-1-receptor antagonist in blocking inflammation mediated by interleukin-1. *N Engl J Med*, 2000, 343, 732-4.

[40] Chazaud, B; Brigitte, M; Yacoub-Youssef, H; Arnold, L; Gherardi, R; Sonnet, C; Lafuste, P; Chretien, F. Dual and beneficial roles of macrophages during skeletal muscle regeneration. *Exerc Sport Sci Rev*, 2009, 37, 18-22.

[41] Gleeson, M. Immune function in sport and exercise. *J Appl Physiol*, 2007, 103, 693-9.

[42] Jonsdottir, IH; Schjerling, P; Ostrowski, K; Asp, S; Richter, EA; Pedersen, BK. Muscle contractions induce interleukin-6 mRNA production in rat skeletal muscles. *J Physiol*, 2000, 528 Pt 1, 157-63.

[43] Starkie, RL; Arkinstall, MJ; Koukoulas, I; Hawley, JA; Febbraio, MA. Carbohydrate ingestion attenuates the increase in plasma interleukin-6, but not skeletal muscle interleukin-6 mRNA, during exercise in humans. *J Physiol*, 2001, 533, 585-91.

[44] Steensberg, A; van Hall, G; Osada, T; Sacchetti, M; Saltin, B; Klarlund Pedersen, B. Production of interleukin-6 in contracting human skeletal muscles can account for the exercise-induced increase in plasma interleukin-6. *J Physiol*, 2000, 529 Pt 1, 237-42.

[45] Weigert, C; Dufer, M; Simon, P; Debre, E; Runge, H; Brodbeck, K; Haring, HU; Schleicher, ED. Upregulation of IL-6 mRNA by IL-6 in skeletal

muscle cells: role of IL-6 mRNA stabilization and Ca2+-dependent mechanisms. *Am J Physiol Cell Physiol*, 2007, 293, C1139-47.

[46] Glund, S; Deshmukh, A; Long, YC; Moller, T; Koistinen, HA; Caidahl, K; Zierath, JR; Krook, A. Interleukin-6 directly increases glucose metabolism in resting human skeletal muscle. *Diabetes*, 2007, 56, 1630-7.

[47] Carey, AL; Steinberg, GR; Macaulay, SL; Thomas, WG; Holmes, AG; Ramm, G; Prelovsek, O; Hohnen-Behrens, C; Watt, MJ; James, DE; Kemp, BE; Pedersen, BK; Febbraio, MA. Interleukin-6 increases insulin-stimulated glucose disposal in humans and glucose uptake and fatty acid oxidation *in vitro* via AMP-activated protein kinase. *Diabetes*, 2006, 55, 2688-97.

[48] Keller, P; Penkowa, M; Keller, C; Steensberg, A; Fischer, CP; Giralt, M; Hidalgo, J; Pedersen, BK. Interleukin-6 receptor expression in contracting human skeletal muscle: regulating role of IL-6. *Faseb J*, 2005, 19, 1181-3.

[49] Wilund, KR. Is the anti-inflammatory effect of regular exercise responsible for reduced cardiovascular disease? *Clin Sci (Lond)*, 2007, 112, 543-55.

[50] Mathur, N; Pedersen, BK. Exercise as a mean to control low-grade systemic inflammation. *Mediators Inflamm*, 2008, Article identification 109502.

[51] Hotamisligil, GS. Inflammation and metabolic disorders. *Nature*, 2006, 444, 860-7.

[52] Haffner, SM. The metabolic syndrome: inflammation, diabetes mellitus, and cardiovascular disease. *Am J Cardiol*, 2006, 97, 3A-11A.

[53] Lin, WW; Karin, M. A cytokine-mediated link between innate immunity, inflammation, and cancer. *J Clin Invest*, 2007, 117, 1175-83.

[54] Roubenoff, R. Physical activity, inflammation, and muscle loss. *Nutr Rev*, 2007, 65, S208-12.

[55] Eid, AA; Ionescu, AA; Nixon, LS; Lewis-Jenkins, V; Matthews, SB; Griffiths, TL; Shale, DJ. Inflammatory response and body composition in chronic obstructive pulmonary disease. *Am J Respir Crit Care Med*, 2001, 164, 1414-8.

[56] Brennan, FM; Maini, RN; Feldmann, M. TNF alpha--a pivotal role in rheumatoid arthritis? *Br J Rheumatol*, 1992, 31, 293-8.

[57] Palacio, J; Galdiz, JB; Bech, JJ; Marinan, M; Casadevall, C; Martinez, P; Gea, J.Interleukin 10 and tumor necrosis factor alpha gene expression in respiratory and peripheral muscles. Relation to sarcolemmal damage. *Arch Bronconeumol*, 2002, 38, 311-6.

[58] Haddad, F; Zaldivar, F; Cooper, DM; Adams, GR. IL-6-induced skeletal muscle atrophy. *J Appl Physiol*, 2005, 98, 911-7.

[59] Coletti, D; Moresi, V; Adamo, S; Molinaro, M; Sassoon, D. Tumor necrosis factor-alpha gene transfer induces cachexia and inhibits muscle regeneration. *Genesis*, 2005, 43, 120-8.

[60] Handschin, C; Spiegelman, B. The role of exercise and PGC1α in inflammation and chronic disease. *Nature*, 2008, 454, 463-469.

[61] Cesari, M; Penninx, BW; Newman, AB; Kritchevsky, SB; Nicklas, BJ; Sutton-Tyrrell, K; Rubin, SM; Ding, J; Simonsick, EM; Harris, TB; Pahor, M. Inflammatory markers and onset of cardiovascular events: results from the Health ABC study. *Circulation*, 2003, 108, 2317-22.

[62] Meyerhardt, JA; Heseltine, D; Niedzwiecki, D; Hollis, D; Saltz, LB; Mayer, RJ; Thomas, J; Nelson, H; Whittom, R; Hantel, A; Schilsky, RL; Fuchs, CS. Impact of physical activity on cancer recurrence and survival in patients with stage III colon cancer: findings from CALGB 89803. *J Clin Oncol*, 2006, 24, 3535-41.

[63] Packard, RR; Libby, P. Inflammation in atherosclerosis: from vascular biology to biomarker discovery and risk prediction. *Clin Chem*, 2008, 54, 24-38.

[64] Plomgaard, P; Bouzakri, K; Krogh-Madsen, R; Mittendorfer, B; Zierath, JR; Pedersen, BK. Tumor necrosis factor-alpha induces skeletal muscle insulin resistance in healthy human subjects via inhibition of Akt substrate 160 phosphorylation. *Diabetes*, 2005, 54, 2939-45.

[65] Hotamisligil, GS; Shargill, NS; Spiegelman, BM. Adipose expression of tumor necrosis factor-alpha: direct role in obesity-linked insulin resistance. *Science*, 1993, 259, 87-91.

[66] Plomgaard, P; Nielsen, AR; Fischer, CP; Mortensen, OH; Broholm, C; Penkowa, M; Krogh-Madsen, R; Erikstrup, C; Lindegaard, B; Petersen, AM; Taudorf, S; Pedersen, BK. Associations between insulin resistance and TNF-alpha in plasma, skeletal muscle and adipose tissue in humans with and without type 2 diabetes. *Diabetologia*, 2007, 50, 2562-71.

[67] Hotamisligil, GS; Arner, P; Caro, JF; Atkinson, RL; Spiegelman, BM. Increased adipose tissue expression of tumor necrosis factor-alpha in human obesity and insulin resistance. *J Clin Invest*, 1995, 95, 2409-15.

[68] Pedersen, BK; Febbraio, MA. Point: Interleukin-6 does have a beneficial role in insulin sensitivity and glucose homeostasis. *J Appl Physiol*, 2007, 102, 814-6.

[69] Steensberg, A; Fischer, CP; Sacchetti, M; Keller, C; Osada, T; Schjerling, P; van Hall, G; Febbraio, MA; Pedersen, BK. Acute interleukin-6 administration does not impair muscle glucose uptake or whole-body glucose disposal in healthy humans. *J Physiol*, 2003, 548, 631-8.

[70] Lyngso, D; Simonsen, L; Bulow, J. Interleukin-6 production in human subcutaneous abdominal adipose tissue: the effect of exercise. *J Physiol*, 2002, 543, 373-8.

[71] Petersen, EW; Carey, AL; Sacchetti, M; Steinberg, GR; Macaulay, SL; Febbraio, MA; Pedersen, BK. Acute IL-6 treatment increases fatty acid turnover in elderly humans *in vivo* and in tissue culture *in vitro*. *Am J Physiol Endocrinol Metab*, 2005, 288, E155-62.

[72] van Hall, G; Steensberg, A; Sacchetti, M; Fischer, C; Keller, C; Schjerling, P; Hiscock, N; Moller, K; Saltin, B; Febbraio, MA; Pedersen, BK. Interleukin-6 stimulates lipolysis and fat oxidation in humans. *J Clin Endocrinol Metab*, 2003, 88, 3005-10.

[73] Nishimoto, N; Yoshizaki, K; Miyasaka, N; Yamamoto, K; Kawai, S; Takeuchi, T; Hashimoto, J; Azuma, J; Kishimoto, T. Treatment of rheumatoid arthritis with humanized anti-interleukin-6 receptor antibody: a multicenter, double-blind, placebo-controlled trial. *Arthritis Rheum*, 2004, 50, 1761-9.

[74] Choy, EH; Isenberg, DA; Garrood, T; Farrow, S; Ioannou, Y; Bird, H; Cheung, N; Williams, B; Hazleman, B; Price, R; Yoshizaki, K; Nishimoto, N; Kishimoto, T; Panayi, GS. Therapeutic benefit of blocking interleukin-6 activity with an anti-interleukin-6 receptor monoclonal antibody in rheumatoid arthritis: a randomized, double-blind, placebo-controlled, dose-escalation trial. *Arthritis Rheum*, 2002, 46, 3143-50.

[75] Coussens, LM; Werb, Z. Inflammation and cancer. *Nature*, 2002, 420, 860-7.

[76] Balkwill, F; Mantovani, A. Inflammation and cancer: back to Virchow? *Lancet*, 2001, 357, 539-45.

[77] Lu, H; Ouyang, W; Huang, C. Inflammation, a key event in cancer development. *Mol Cancer Res*, 2006, 4, 221-33.

[78] Itzkowitz, SH; Yio, X. Inflammation and cancer IV. Colorectal cancer in inflammatory bowel disease: the role of inflammation. *Am J Physiol Gastrointest Liver Physiol*, 2004, 287, G7-17.

[79] Seril, DN; Liao, J; Yang, GY; Yang, CS. Oxidative stress and ulcerative colitis-associated carcinogenesis: studies in humans and animal models. *Carcinogenesis*, 2003, 24, 353-62.

[80] Moody, GA; Jayanthi, V; Probert, CS; Mac Kay, H; Mayberry, JF. Long-term therapy with sulphasalazine protects against colorectal cancer in ulcerative colitis: a retrospective study of colorectal cancer risk and compliance with treatment in Leicestershire. *Eur J Gastroenterol Hepatol*, 1996, 8, 1179-83.

[81] Eaden, J; Abrams, K; Ekbom, A; Jackson, E; Mayberry, J. Colorectal cancer prevention in ulcerative colitis: a case-control study. *Aliment Pharmacol Ther*, 2000, 14, 145-53.

[82] Thun, MJ; Namboodiri, MM; Calle, EE; Flanders, WD; Heath, CW, Jr. Aspirin use and risk of fatal cancer. *Cancer Res*, 1993, 53, 1322-7.

[83] Langman, MJ; Cheng, KK; Gilman, EA; Lancashire, RJ. Effect of anti-inflammatory drugs on overall risk of common cancer: case-control study in general practice research database. *Bmj*, 2000, 320, 1642-6.

[84] Moore, RJ; Owens, DM; Stamp, G; Arnott, C; Burke, F; East, N; Holdsworth, H; Turner, L; Rollins, B; Pasparakis, M; Kollias, G; Balkwill, F. Mice deficient in tumor necrosis factor-alpha are resistant to skin carcinogenesis. *Nat Med*, 1999, 5, 828-31.

[85] Karin, M. Nuclear factor-kappaB in cancer development and progression. *Nature*, 2006, 441, 431-6.

[86] Febbraio, MA. Exercise and inflammation. *J Appl Physiol*, 2007, 103, 376-7.

[87] Nieman, DC. Current perspective on exercise immunology. *Curr Sports Med Rep*, 2003, 2, 239-42.

[88] Gleeson, M; McFarlin, B; Flynn, M. Exercise and Toll-like receptors. *Exerc Immunol Rev*, 2006, 12, 34-53.

[89] Gleeson, M; Nieman, DC; Pedersen, BK. Exercise, nutrition and immune function. *J Sports Sci*, 2004, 22, 115-25.

[90] Cannon, J; Blumberg, JB. Acute phase immune response in exercise. In: Sen CK, Packer L, Hänninen O, eds. Handbook of Oxidants and Antioxidants in Exercise. Amsterdam: Elsevier Science B.V., 2000:177-194.

[91] Pizza, FX; Davis, BH; Henrickson, SD; Mitchell, JB; Pace, JF; Bigelow, N; DiLauro, P; Naglieri, T. Adaptation to eccentric exercise: effect on CD64 and CD11b/CD18 expression. *J Appl Physiol*, 1996, 80, 47-55.

[92] Tidball, JG. Inflammatory cell response to acute muscle injury. *Med Sci Sports Exerc*, 1995, 27, 1022-32.

[93] Nieman, DC. Exercise immunology: integration and regulation. *Int J Sports Med*, 1998, 19 Suppl 3, S171.

[94] Tauler, P; Aguilo, A; Gimeno, I; Noguera, A; Agusti, A; Tur, JA; Pons, A. Differential response of lymphocytes and neutrophils to high intensity physical activity and to vitamin C diet supplementation. *Free Radic Res*, 2003, 37, 931-8.

[95] Tauler, P; Aguilo, A; Gimeno, I; Guix, P; Tur, JA; Pons, A. Different effects of exercise tests on the antioxidant enzyme activities in lymphocytes and neutrophils. *J Nutr Biochem*, 2004, 15, 479-84.

[96] Hessel, E; Haberland, A; Muller, M; Lerche, D; Schimke, I. Oxygen radical generation of neutrophils: a reason for oxidative stress during marathon running? *Clin Chim Acta*, 2000, 298, 145-56.

[97] McCarthy, DA; Dale, MM. The leucocytosis of exercise. A review and model. *Sports Med*, 1988, 6, 333-63.

[98] Pedersen, BK; Hoffman-Goetz, L. Exercise and the immune system: regulation, integration, and adaptation. *Physiol Rev*, 2000, 80, 1055-81.

[99] Nieman, DC; Johanssen, LM; Lee, JW; Arabatzis, K. Infectious episodes in runners before and after the Los Angeles Marathon. *J Sports Med Phys Fitness*, 1990, 30, 316-28.

[100] Peters, EM; Bateman, ED. Ultramarathon running and upper respiratory tract infections. An epidemiological survey. *S Afr Med J*, 1983, 64, 582-4.

[101] Peters, EM; Goetzsche, JM; Grobbelaar, B; Noakes, TD. Vitamin C supplementation reduces the incidence of post-trace symptoms of upper-respiratory-tract infection in ultramarathon runners. *Am J Clin Nutr*, 1993, 57, 170-4.

[102] Nieman, DC. Exercise, upper respiratory tract infection, and the immune system. *Med Sci Sports Exerc*, 1994, 26, 128-39.

[103] Pedersen, BK; Nieman, DC. Exercise immunology: integration and regulation. *Immunol Today*, 1998, 19, 204-6.

[104] Febbraio, MA; Pedersen, BK. Muscle-derived interleukin-6: mechanisms for activation and possible biological roles. *Faseb J*, 2002, 16, 1335-47.

[105] Ostrowski, K; Rohde, T; Asp, S; Schjerling, P; Pedersen, BK. Pro- and anti-inflammatory cytokine balance in strenuous exercise in humans. *J Physiol*, 1999, 515 (Pt 1), 287-91.

[106] Pedersen, BK; Steensberg, A; Schjerling, P. Muscle-derived interleukin-6: possible biological effects. *J Physiol*, 2001, 536, 329-37.

[107] Ostrowski, K; Schjerling, P; Pedersen, BK. Physical activity and plasma interleukin-6 in humans--effect of intensity of exercise. *Eur J Appl Physiol*, 2000, 83, 512-5.

[108] Pedersen, BK; Steensberg, A; Schjerling, P. Exercise and interleukin-6. *Curr Opin Hematol*, 2001, 8, 137-41.

[109] Pedersen, BK. IL-6 signaling in exercise and disease. *Biochem Soc Trans*, 2007, 35, 1295-7.

[110] Ostrowski, K; Rohde, T; Asp, S; Schjerling, P; Pedersen, BK. Chemokines are elevated in plasma after strenuous exercise in humans. *Eur J Appl Physiol*, 2001, 84, 244-5.

[111] Nieman, DC; Davis, JM; Henson, DA; Walberg-Rankin, J; Shute, M; Dumke, CL; Utter, AC; Vinci, DM; Carson, JA; Brown, A; Lee, WJ; McAnulty, SR; McAnulty, LS. Carbohydrate ingestion influences skeletal muscle cytokine mRNA and plasma cytokine levels after a 3-h run. *J Appl Physiol*, 2003, 94, 1917-25.

[112] Chan, MH; Carey, AL; Watt, MJ; Febbraio, MA. Cytokine gene expression in human skeletal muscle during concentric contraction: evidence that IL-8, like IL-6, is influenced by glycogen availability. *Am J Physiol Regul Integr Comp Physiol*, 2004, 287, R322-7.

[113] Henson, DA; Nieman, DC; Nehlsen-Cannarella, SL; Fagoaga, OR; Shannon, M; Bolton, MR; Davis, JM; Gaffney, CT; Kelln, WJ; Austin, MD; Hjertman, JM; Schilling, BK. Influence of carbohydrate on cytokine and phagocytic responses to 2 h of rowing. *Med Sci Sports Exerc*, 2000, 32, 1384-9.

[114] Akerstrom, T; Steensberg, A; Keller, P; Keller, C; Penkowa, M; Pedersen, BK. Exercise induces interleukin-8 expression in human skeletal muscle. *J Physiol*, 2005, 563, 507-16.

[115] De Rossi, M; Bernasconi, P; Baggi, F; de Waal Malefyt, R; Mantegazza, R. Cytokines and chemokines are both expressed by human myoblasts: possible relevance for the immune pathogenesis of muscle inflammation. *Int Immunol*, 2000, 12, 1329-35.

[116] Baggiolini, M. Chemokines in pathology and medicine. *J Intern Med*, 2001, 250, 91-104.

[117] Nielsen, AR; Mounier, R; Plomgaard, P; Mortensen, OH; Penkowa, M; Speerschneider, T; Pilegaard, H; Pedersen, BK. Expression of interleukin-15 in human skeletal muscle effect of exercise and muscle fibre type composition. *J Physiol*, 2007, 584, 305-12.

[118] Riechman, SE; Balasekaran, G; Roth, SM; Ferrell, RE. Association of interleukin-15 protein and interleukin-15 receptor genetic variation with resistance exercise training responses. *J Appl Physiol*, 2004, 97, 2214-9.

[119] Nieman, DC; Davis, JM; Brown, VA; Henson, DA; Dumke, CL; Utter, AC; Vinci, DM; Downs, MF; Smith, JC; Carson, J; Brown, A; McAnulty, SR; McAnulty, LS. Influence of carbohydrate ingestion on immune changes after 2 h of intensive resistance training. *J Appl Physiol*, 2004, 96, 1292-8.

[120] Grabstein, KH; Eisenman, J; Shanebeck, K; Rauch, C; Srinivasan, S; Fung, V; Beers, C; Richardson, J; Schoenborn, MA; Ahdieh, M; *et al.* Cloning of

a T cell growth factor that interacts with the beta chain of the interleukin-2 receptor. *Science*, 1994, 264, 965-8.

[121] Argiles, JM; Lopez-Soriano, J; Almendro, V; Busquets, S; Lopez-Soriano, FJ. Cross-talk between skeletal muscle and adipose tissue: a link with obesity? *Med Res Rev*, 2005, 25, 49-65.

[122] Weight, LM; Alexander, D; Jacobs, P. Strenuous exercise: analogous to the acute-phase response? *Clin Sci (Lond)*, 1991, 81, 677-83.

[123] Das, UN. Anti-inflammatory nature of exercise. *Nutrition*, 2004, 20, 323-6.

[124] Niess, AM; Passek, F; Lorenz, I; Schneider, EM; Dickhuth, HH; Northoff, H; Fehrenbach, E. Expression of the antioxidant stress protein heme oxygenase-1 (HO-1) in human leukocytes. *Free Radic Biol Med*, 1999, 26, 184-92.

[125] Thompson, D; Basu-Modak, S; Gordon, M; Poore, S; Markovitch, D; Tyrrell, RM. Exercise-induced expression of heme oxygenase-1 in human lymphocytes. *Free Radic Res*, 2005, 39, 63-9.

[126] Pedersen, M; Steensberg, A; Keller, C; Osada, T; Zacho, M; Saltin, B; Febbraio, MA; Pedersen, BK. Does the aging skeletal muscle maintain its endocrine function? *Exerc Immunol Rev*, 2004, 10, 42-55.

[127] Fischer, CP; Hiscock, NJ; Penkowa, M; Basu, S; Vessby, B; Kallner, A; Sjoberg, LB; Pedersen, BK. Supplementation with vitamins C and E inhibits the release of interleukin-6 from contracting human skeletal muscle. *J Physiol*, 2004, 558, 633-45.

[128] Ostrowski, K; Rohde, T; Zacho, M; Asp, S; Pedersen, BK. Evidence that interleukin-6 is produced in human skeletal muscle during prolonged running. *J Physiol*, 1998, 508 (Pt 3), 949-53.

[129] Steensberg, A; Febbraio, MA; Osada, T; Schjerling, P; van Hall, G; Saltin, B; Pedersen, BK. Interleukin-6 production in contracting human skeletal muscle is influenced by pre-exercise muscle glycogen content. *J Physiol*, 2001, 537, 633-9.

[130] Steensberg, A; Keller, C; Starkie, RL; Osada, T; Febbraio, MA; Pedersen, BK. IL-6 and TNF-alpha expression in, and release from, contracting human skeletal muscle. *Am J Physiol Endocrinol Metab*, 2002, 283, E1272-8.

[131] Febbraio, MA; Steensberg, A; Keller, C; Starkie, RL; Nielsen, HB; Krustrup, P; Ott, P; Secher, NH; Pedersen, BK. Glucose ingestion attenuates interleukin-6 release from contracting skeletal muscle in humans. *J Physiol*, 2003, 549, 607-12.

[132] Pedersen, BK; Akerstrom, TC; Nielsen, AR; Fischer, CP. Role of myokines in exercise and metabolism. *J Appl Physiol*, 2007, 103, 1093-8.

[133] Keller, C; Steensberg, A; Pilegaard, H; Osada, T; Saltin, B; Pedersen, BK; Neufer, PD. Transcriptional activation of the IL-6 gene in human contracting skeletal muscle: influence of muscle glycogen content. *Faseb J*, 2001, 15, 2748-50.

[134] Hiscock, N; Chan, MH; Bisucci, T; Darby, IA; Febbraio, MA. Skeletal myocytes are a source of interleukin-6 mRNA expression and protein release during contraction: evidence of fiber type specificity. *Faseb J*, 2004, 18, 992-4.

[135] Steensberg, A; Keller, C; Hillig, T; Frosig, C; Wojtaszewski, JF; Pedersen, BK; Pilegaard, H; Sander, M. Nitric oxide production is a proximal signaling event controlling exercise-induced mRNA expression in human skeletal muscle. *Faseb J*, 2007, 21, 2683-94.

[136] Keller, C; Hellsten, Y; Steensberg, A; Pedersen, BK. Differential regulation of IL-6 and TNF-alpha via calcineurin in human skeletal muscle cells. *Cytokine*, 2006, 36, 141-7.

[137] Chan, MH; McGee, SL; Watt, MJ; Hargreaves, M; Febbraio, MA. Altering dietary nutrient intake that reduces glycogen content leads to phosphorylation of nuclear p38 MAP kinase in human skeletal muscle: association with IL-6 gene transcription during contraction. *Faseb J*, 2004, 18, 1785-7.

[138] Pedersen, BK. The anti-inflammatory effect of exercise: its role in diabetes and cardiovascular disease control. *Essays Biochem*, 2006, 42, 105-17.

[139] Steensberg, A; Fischer, CP; Keller, C; Moller, K; Pedersen, BK. IL-6 enhances plasma IL-1ra, IL-10, and cortisol in humans. *Am J Physiol Endocrinol Metab*, 2003, 285, E433-7.

[140] Schindler, R; Mancilla, J; Endres, S; Ghorbani, R; Clark, SC; Dinarello, CA. Correlations and interactions in the production of interleukin-6 (IL-6), IL-1, and tumor necrosis factor (TNF) in human blood mononuclear cells: IL-6 suppresses IL-1 and TNF. *Blood*, 1990, 75, 40-7.

[141] Starkie, R; Ostrowski, SR; Jauffred, S; Febbraio, M; Pedersen, BK. Exercise and IL-6 infusion inhibit endotoxin-induced TNF-alpha production in humans. *Faseb J*, 2003, 17, 884-6.

[142] Fiers, W. Tumor necrosis factor. Characterization at the molecular, cellular and in vivo level. *FEBS Lett*, 1991, 285, 199-212.

[143] Matthys, P; Mitera, T; Heremans, H; Van Damme, J; Billiau, A. Anti-gamma interferon and anti-interleukin-6 antibodies affect staphylococcal enterotoxin B-induced weight loss, hypoglycemia, and cytokine release in D-galactosamine-sensitized and unsensitized mice. *Infect Immun*, 1995, 63, 1158-64.

[144] Mizuhara, H; O'Neill, E; Seki, N; Ogawa, T; Kusunoki, C; Otsuka, K; Satoh, S; Niwa, M; Senoh, H; Fujiwara, H. T cell activation-associated hepatic injury: mediation by tumor necrosis factors and protection by interleukin 6. *J Exp Med*, 1994, 179, 1529-37.

[145] Pretolani, M. Interleukin-10: an anti-inflammatory cytokine with therapeutic potential. *Clin Exp Allergy*, 1999, 29, 1164–1171.

[146] Pue, C; Mortensen, R; Marsh, C; Pope, H; Wewers, M. Acute phase levels of C-reactive protein enhance IL-1 beta and IL-1ra production by human blood monocytes but inhibit IL-1 beta and IL-1ra production by alveolar macrophages. *J Immunol*, 1996, 156, 1594–1600.

[147] Keller, C; Keller, P; Giralt, M; Hidalgo, J; Pedersen, BK. Exercise normalizes overexpression of TNF-alpha in knockout mice. *Biochem Biophys Res Commun*, 2004, 321, 179-82.

[148] van der Poll, T; Coyle, SM; Barbosa, K; Braxton, CC; Lowry, SF. Epinephrine inhibits tumor necrosis factor-alpha and potentiates interleukin 10 production during human endotoxemia. *J Clin Invest*, 1996, 97, 713-9.

[149] Steensberg, A; Toft, AD; Schjerling, P; Halkjaer-Kristensen, J; Pedersen, BK. Plasma interleukin-6 during strenuous exercise: role of epinephrine. *Am J Physiol Cell Physiol*, 2001, 281, C1001-4.

[150] Nieman, DC; Henson, DA; Austin, MD; Brown, VA. Immune response to a 30-minute walk. *Med Sci Sports Exerc*, 2005, 37, 57-62.

[151] Plaisance, EP; Taylor, JK; Alhassan, S; Abebe, A; Mestek, ML; Grandjean, PW. Cardiovascular fitness and vascular inflammatory markers after acute aerobic exercise. *Int J Sport Nutr Exerc Metab*, 2007, 17, 152-62.

[152] Mills, PJ; Maisel, AS; Ziegler, MG; Dimsdale, JE; Carter, S; Kennedy, B; Woods, VL, Jr. Peripheral blood mononuclear cell-endothelial adhesion in human hypertension following exercise. *J Hypertens*, 2000, 18, 1801-6.

[153] Peake, JM; Suzuki, K; Hordern, M; Wilson, G; Nosaka, K; Coombes, JS. Plasma cytokine changes in relation to exercise intensity and muscle damage. *Eur J Appl Physiol*, 2005, 95, 514-21.

[154] Markovitch, D; Tyrrell, RM; Thompson, D. Acute moderate-intensity exercise in middle-aged men has neither an anti- nor proinflammatory effect. *J Appl Physiol*, 2008, 105, 260-5.

[155] Steinberg, JG; Ba, A; Bregeon, F; Delliaux, S; Jammes, Y. Cytokine and oxidative responses to maximal cycling exercise in sedentary subjects. *Med Sci Sports Exerc*, 2007, 39, 964-8.

[156] Zaldivar, F; Wang-Rodriguez, J; Nemet, D; Schwindt, C; Galassetti, P; Mills, PJ; Wilson, LD; Cooper, DM. Constitutive pro- and anti-

inflammatory cytokine and growth factor response to exercise in leukocytes. *J Appl Physiol*, 2006, 100, 1124-33.

[157] Li, YP; Reid, MB. Effect of tumor necrosis factor-alpha on skeletal muscle metabolism. *Curr Opin Rheumatol*, 2001, 13, 483-7.

[158] Plaisance, EP; Grandjean, PW. Physical activity and high-sensitivity C-reactive protein. *Sports Med*, 2006, 36, 443-58.

[159] Bruunsgaard, H. Physical activity and modulation of systemic low-level inflammation. *J Leukoc Biol*, 2005, 78, 819-35.

[160] Smith, JK; Dykes, R; Douglas, JE; Krishnaswamy, G; Berk, S. Long-term exercise and atherogenic activity of blood mononuclear cells in persons at risk of developing ischemic heart disease. *Jama*, 1999, 281, 1722-7.

[161] Sanders, AE; Slade, GD; Fitzsimmons, TR; Bartold, PM. Physical activity, inflammatory biomarkers in gingival crevicular fluid and periodontitis. *J Clin Periodontol*, 2009, 36, 388-95.

[162] Fallon, KE; Fallon, SK; Boston, T. The acute phase response and exercise: court and field sports. *Br J Sports Med*, 2001, 35, 170-3.

[163] Mattusch, F; Dufaux, B; Heine, O; Mertens, I; Rost, R. Reduction of the plasma concentration of C-reactive protein following nine months of endurance training. *Int J Sports Med*, 2000, 21, 21-4.

[164] Abramson, JL; Vaccarino, V. Relationship between physical activity and inflammation among apparently healthy middle-aged and older US adults. *Arch Intern Med*, 2002, 162, 1286-92.

[165] Geffken, DF; Cushman, M; Burke, GL; Polak, JF; Sakkinen, PA; Tracy, RP. Association between physical activity and markers of inflammation in a healthy elderly population. *Am J Epidemiol*, 2001, 153, 242-50.

[166] King, DE; Carek, P; Mainous, AG, 3rd; Pearson, WS. Inflammatory markers and exercise: differences related to exercise type. *Med Sci Sports Exerc*, 2003, 35, 575-81.

[167] Taaffe, DR; Harris, TB; Ferrucci, L; Rowe, J; Seeman, TE. Cross-sectional and prospective relationships of interleukin-6 and C-reactive protein with physical performance in elderly persons: MacArthur studies of successful aging. *J Gerontol A Biol Sci Med Sci*, 2000, 55, M709-15.

[168] Wannamethee, SG; Lowe, GD; Whincup, PH; Rumley, A; Walker, M; Lennon, L. Physical activity and hemostatic and inflammatory variables in elderly men. *Circulation*, 2002, 105, 1785-90.

[169] Bruunsgaard, H; Ladelund, S; Pedersen, AN; Schroll, M; Jorgensen, T; Pedersen, BK. Predicting death from tumor necrosis factor-alpha and interleukin-6 in 80-year-old people. *Clin Exp Immunol*, 2003, 132, 24-31.

[170] Tisi, PV; Hulse, M; Chulakadabba, A; Gosling, P; Shearman, CP. Exercise training for intermittent claudication: does it adversely affect biochemical markers of the exercise-induced inflammatory response? *Eur J Vasc Endovasc Surg*, 1997, 14, 344-50.

[171] Stewart, LK; Flynn, MG; Campbell, WW; Craig, BA; Robinson, JP; Timmerman, KL; McFarlin, BK; Coen, PM; Talbert, E. The influence of exercise training on inflammatory cytokines and C-reactive protein. *Med Sci Sports Exerc*, 2007, 39, 1714-9.

[172] Goldhammer, E; Tanchilevitch, A; Maor, I; Beniamini, Y; Rosenschein, U; Sagiv, M. Exercise training modulates cytokines activity in coronary heart disease patients. *Int J Cardiol*, 2005, 100, 93-9.

[173] Kelley, GA; Kelley, KS. Effects of aerobic exercise on C-reactive protein, body composition, and maximum oxygen consumption in adults: a meta-analysis of randomized controlled trials. *Metabolism*, 2006, 55, 1500-7.

[174] Kohut, ML; McCann, DA; Russell, DW; Konopka, DN; Cunnick, JE; Franke, WD; Castillo, MC; Reighard, AE; Vanderah, E. Aerobic exercise, but not flexibility/resistance exercise, reduces serum IL-18, CRP, and IL-6 independent of beta-blockers, BMI, and psychosocial factors in older adults. *Brain Behav Immun*, 2006, 20, 201-9.

[175] Ford, ES. Does exercise reduce inflammation? Physical activity and C-reactive protein among U.S. adults. *Epidemiology*, 2002, 13, 561-8.

[176] Fischer, CP; Berntsen, A; Perstrup, LB; Eskildsen, P; Pedersen, BK. Plasma levels of interleukin-6 and C-reactive protein are associated with physical inactivity independent of obesity. *Scand J Med Sci Sports*, 2007, 17, 580-7.

[177] Mora, S; Lee, IM; Buring, JE; Ridker, PM. Association of physical activity and body mass index with novel and traditional cardiovascular biomarkers in women. *Jama*, 2006, 295, 1412-9.

[178] Kasapis, C; Thompson, PD. The effects of physical activity on serum C-reactive protein and inflammatory markers: a systematic review. *J Am Coll Cardiol*, 2005, 45, 1563-9.

[179] Dufaux, B; Order, U; Geyer, H; Hollmann, W. C-reactive protein serum concentrations in well-trained athletes. *Int J Sports Med*, 1984, 5, 102-6.

[180] Rauramaa, R; Halonen, P; Vaisanen, SB; Lakka, TA; Schmidt-Trucksass, A; Berg, A; Penttila, IM; Rankinen, T; Bouchard, C. Effects of aerobic physical exercise on inflammation and atherosclerosis in men: the DNASCO Study: a six-year randomized, controlled trial. *Ann Intern Med*, 2004, 140, 1007-14.

[181] Verdaet, D; Dendale, P; De Bacquer, D; Delanghe, J; Block, P; De Backer, G. Association between leisure time physical activity and markers of

chronic inflammation related to coronary heart disease. *Atherosclerosis,* 2004, 176, 303-10.

[182] Rawson, ES; Freedson, PS; Osganian, SK; Matthews, CE; Reed, G; Ockene, IS. Body mass index, but not physical activity, is associated with C-reactive protein. *Med Sci Sports Exerc,* 2003, 35, 1160-6.

[183] Arsenault, BJ; Cartier, A; Cote, M; Lemieux, I; Tremblay, A; Bouchard, C; Perusse, L; Despres, JP. Body composition, cardiorespiratory fitness, and low-grade inflammation in middle-aged men and women. *Am J Cardiol,* 2009, 104, 240-6.

[184] Selvin, E; Paynter, NP; Erlinger, TP. The effect of weight loss on C-reactive protein: a systematic review. *Arch Intern Med,* 2007, 167, 31-9.

[185] Kondo, N; Nomura, M; Nakaya, Y; Ito, S; Ohguro, T. Association of inflammatory marker and highly sensitive C-reactive protein with aerobic exercise capacity, maximum oxygen uptake and insulin resistance in healthy middle-aged volunteers. *Circ J,* 2005, 69, 452-7.

[186] Jankord, R; Jemiolo, B. Influence of physical activity on serum IL-6 and IL-10 levels in healthy older men. *Med Sci Sports Exerc,* 2004, 36, 960-4.

[187] Colbert, LH; Visser, M; Simonsick, EM; Tracy, RP; Newman, AB; Kritchevsky, SB; Pahor, M; Taaffe, DR; Brach, J; Rubin, S; Harris, TB. Physical activity, exercise, and inflammatory markers in older adults: findings from the Health, Aging and Body Composition Study. *J Am Geriatr Soc,* 2004, 52, 1098-104.

[188] Hammett, CJ; Prapavessis, H; Baldi, JC; Varo, N; Schoenbeck, U; Ameratunga, R; French, JK; White, HD; Stewart, RA. Effects of exercise training on 5 inflammatory markers associated with cardiovascular risk. *Am Heart J,* 2006, 151, 367 e7-367 e16.

[189] Sloan, RP; Shapiro, PA; Demeersman, RE; McKinley, PS; Tracey, KJ; Slavov, I; Fang, Y; Flood, PD. Aerobic exercise attenuates inducible TNF production in humans. *J Appl Physiol,* 2007, 103, 1007-11.

[190] Albert, MA; Glynn, RJ; Ridker, PM. Effect of physical activity on serum C-reactive protein. *Am J Cardiol,* 2004, 93, 221-5.

[191] Isasi, CR; Deckelbaum, RJ; Tracy, RP; Starc, TJ; Berglund, L; Shea, S. Physical fitness and C-reactive protein level in children and young adults: the Columbia University BioMarkers Study. *Pediatrics,* 2003, 111, 332-8.

[192] Hardman, AE. The influence of exercise on postprandial triacylglycerol metabolism. *Atherosclerosis,* 1998, 141 Suppl 1, S93-100.

[193] LaMonte, MJ; Durstine, JL; Yanowitz, FG; Lim, T; DuBose, KD; Davis, P; Ainsworth, BE. Cardiorespiratory fitness and C-reactive protein among a tri-ethnic sample of women. *Circulation,* 2002, 106, 403-6.

[194] Pitsavos, C; Panagiotakos, DB; Chrysohoou, C; Kavouras, S; Stefanadis, C. The associations between physical activity, inflammation, and coagulation markers, in people with metabolic syndrome: the ATTICA study. *Eur J Cardiovasc Prev Rehabil*, 2005, 12, 151-8.

[195] Okita, K; Nishijima, H; Murakami, T; Nagai, T; Morita, N; Yonezawa, K; Iizuka, K; Kawaguchi, H; Kitabatake, A. Can exercise training with weight loss lower serum C-reactive protein levels? *Arterioscler Thromb Vasc Biol*, 2004, 24, 1868-73.

[196] Nicklas, BJ; Ambrosius, W; Messier, SP; Miller, GD; Penninx, BW; Loeser, RF; Palla, S; Bleecker, E; Pahor, M. Diet-induced weight loss, exercise, and chronic inflammation in older, obese adults: a randomized controlled clinical trial. *Am J Clin Nutr*, 2004, 79, 544-51.

[197] Shojaee-Moradie, F; Baynes, KC; Pentecost, C; Bell, JD; Thomas, EL; Jackson, NC; Stolinski, M; Whyte, M; Lovell, D; Bowes, SB; Gibney, J; Jones, RH; Umpleby, AM. Exercise training reduces fatty acid availability and improves the insulin sensitivity of glucose metabolism. *Diabetologia*, 2007, 50, 404-13.

INDEX

A

achievement, 26
acid, 37, 39, 49
activation, 4, 18, 41, 44, 45
activity level, 25
acute infection, 3, 12
adaptation, 11, 41
adhesion, 20, 27, 29, 45
adhesion level, 29
adipose, 8, 15, 26, 35, 38, 39, 43
adipose tissue, 8, 15, 26, 35, 38, 39, 43
adjustment, 8
adrenaline, 12
adults, 25, 46, 47, 49
aerobic exercise, xii, 25, 28, 45, 47, 48
age, 7, 20, 25, 27, 28
aging, 43
allergic reaction, 4
alveolar macrophage, 45
animals, 3, 8
antagonism, 36
antibody, 4, 39
anti-inflammatory agents, 9
anti-inflammatory drugs, 40
antioxidant, 27, 41, 43
apoptosis, 9
artery, 30
atherosclerosis, xi, 1, 2, 8, 29, 35, 38, 47
athletes, 11, 12, 47
atrophy, 7, 37

B

beneficial effect, xi, 1, 4, 11, 23, 27, 29
biomarkers, 27, 46, 47
blood, 4, 8, 24, 29, 44, 45, 46
blood monocytes, 45
blood stream, 4
body composition, 25, 26, 33, 37, 47
body fat, 26
body mass index (BMI), 1, 25, 26, 33, 34, 37, 47
body weight, 34
brain, 35
breast cancer, xi, 1

C

C reactive protein, 3
Ca^{2+}, 4, 18, 37
cachexia, 15, 23, 38
cancer, 1, 7, 9, 33, 37, 38, 39, 40
carbohydrate, 42
carcinogenesis, 9, 39, 40
cardiovascular disease, xi, 1, 7, 8, 25, 33, 34, 35, 37, 44
cardiovascular risk, 26, 29, 48
catecholamines, 9

causal relationship, 24
cell, 4, 8, 9, 15, 40, 45
cell culture, 9, 15
chemokines, 42
children, 48
cholesterol, 9, 27
chronic diseases, xi, xii, 1, 2, 5, 7, 9, 23, 31
chronic obstructive pulmonary disease, 2, 37
circulation, xi, 12, 13, 17, 18
claudication, xi, 24, 47
clinical trials, 9
coagulation, 49
colitis, 9
colon, xi, 1, 9, 38
colon cancer, xi, 1, 9, 38
colorectal cancer, 9, 39
composition, 42, 48
compounds, 18
concentration, 11, 12, 13, 14, 20, 25, 28, 46
confounders, 8, 25
control, 9, 19, 25, 27, 37, 40, 44
control group, 25
controlled trials, 47
COPD, 2, 7, 8, 23
coronary heart disease, 47, 48
cortisol, 11, 12, 18, 44
CRP, 2, 3, 7, 8, 12, 13, 15, 19, 23, 24, 25, 26, 27, 28, 29, 47
culture, 39
cycling, 28, 34, 45
cytokines, xi, 2, 3, 4, 7, 9, 12, 13, 15, 17, 18, 23, 27, 30, 47

D

database, 40
death, 1, 31, 46
degradation, 15
degradation rate, 15
density, 29
Department of Health and Human Services, 33
depression, 11, 12
diabetes, 1, 8, 9, 25, 33, 34, 35, 37, 44
diet, 40

differentiation, 4, 23
disability, 35
donors, 18
dose-response relationship, 24
down-regulation, 29
duration, 11, 13, 17, 20
dyslipidemia, 29

E

elderly, xi, 24, 27, 34, 35, 39, 46
elderly population, 46
endocrine, 2, 4, 14, 43
endothelial cells, 20
endotoxemia, 19, 45
endurance, 13, 17, 46
environment, 4, 19, 23, 29
eosinophils, 4
epinephrine, 11, 12, 19, 45
etiology, 8
exercise, xi, xii, 1, 4, 11, 12, 13, 14, 15, 17, 18, 19, 20, 23, 24, 25, 26, 27, 28, 29, 31, 33, 35, 36, 37, 38, 39, 40, 41, 42, 43, 44, 45, 46, 47, 48, 49
extensor, 20

F

fat, xii, 8, 15, 26, 29, 39
females, 28
fibers, 14, 17
fibrinogen, 25, 26, 27
fitness, 1, 20, 23, 25, 26, 28, 34, 45, 48
flexibility, 25, 28, 47
fluctuations, 4
fluid, 46
football, 28

G

gender, 26, 28
gender differences, 28
gene, 9, 17, 18, 37, 38, 42, 44
gene expression, 37, 42

gene transfer, 38
generation, 41
genes, 36
glucagon, 9
glucose, 4, 8, 34, 37, 38, 49
glucose tolerance, 34
glycogen, 17, 42, 43, 44
groups, 25
growth, 9, 11, 12, 15, 43, 46
growth factor, 43, 46
growth hormone, 11, 12

H

HDL, 27, 29
health, xi, 1, 35
health status, 35
heart disease, 2, 24, 46
heart failure, 2, 35
heme, 43
heme oxygenase, 43
hepatic injury, 45
high density lipoprotein, 27
HO-1, 17, 20, 29, 43
homeostasis, 38
hormone, 4, 12
host, 7
human neutrophils, 36
human subjects, 38
humoral immunity, 4
hyperlipidemia, 1
hypertension, 1, 25, 45
hypoglycemia, 44
hypothesis, 29

I

identification, 37
IFN, 23
IL-13, 4
IL-6, ix, 3, 4, 7, 8, 12, 13, 15, 17, 18, 19, 20,
    23, 25, 26, 28, 31, 35, 36, 37, 39, 41, 42,
    43, 44, 47, 48
IL-8, 7, 13, 14, 18, 42

immune function, 12, 40
immune response, 4, 11, 40
immune system, 4, 11, 12, 41
immunity, 11
immunocompetent cells, 11
in vitro, 14, 18, 37, 39
in vivo, 8, 19, 39, 44
incidence, 9, 12, 41
inducer, 18
induction, 19
infection, 3, 7, 11, 12, 41
inflammation, xi, 2, 3, 4, 5, 7, 8, 9, 11, 15, 17,
    18, 19, 24, 25, 26, 29, 31, 36, 37, 38, 39,
    40, 42, 46, 47, 48, 49
inflammatory bowel disease, 9, 39
inflammatory disease, 35
ingestion, 36, 42, 43
inhibition, 7, 19, 23, 38
inhibitor, 3, 35
initiation, 9
innate immunity, 37
insulin, xi, 1, 2, 7, 8, 26, 35, 37, 38, 48, 49
insulin resistance, xi, 1, 2, 7, 8, 26, 35, 38, 48
insulin sensitivity, 38, 49
insulin signaling, 8
integration, 40, 41
interaction, 15
interactions, 44
interferon, 44
interleukin-8, 36, 42
intervention, 1, 24, 25, 29

L

LDL, 29
leisure, 34, 47
leisure time, 34, 47
lesions, 30
lipid metabolism, 29
lipids, 15, 34
lipolysis, 9, 39
liver, 3, 15, 35
low-density lipoprotein, 27, 29
low-grade inflammation, xi, xii, 19, 24, 26,
    28, 48

lung disease, 1
lymphocytes, 3, 4, 17, 20, 40, 41, 43

M

macrophage inflammatory protein, 12
macrophages, 4, 14, 18, 30, 36
males, 19, 28
malignancy, 9
measures, 21
mediation, 45
men, 21, 25, 27, 28, 33, 34, 35, 45, 46, 47, 48
meta-analysis, 25, 47
metabolic disorder, 23, 37
metabolic syndrome, 8, 37, 49
metabolism, 4, 8, 23, 37, 43, 46, 48, 49
mice, 9, 19, 44, 45
models, 27, 39
molecules, 4, 29
monoclonal antibody, 39
mortality, 1, 33, 34, 35
mRNA, 8, 14, 17, 18, 36, 42, 44
muscle mass, 13, 17
muscle strength, 23
muscles, 14, 17, 31, 37
myoblasts, 42

N

necrosis, 38, 44
network, 18
neutrophils, 3, 14, 18, 40, 41
nitric oxide, 18
non-steroidal anti-inflammatory drugs, 9
nutrition, 40

O

obesity, 1, 7, 8, 27, 35, 38, 43, 47
older adults, 47, 48
organ, 2, 4
oxidation, 8, 30, 37, 39
oxidative stress, 41
oxygen, 47, 48

oxygen consumption, 47

P

pathogenesis, 2, 7, 42
pathogens, 4
pathology, 42
pathways, 18, 19, 29
periodontitis, 24, 46
peripheral blood, 36
peripheral blood mononuclear cell, 36
phosphorylation, 38, 44
physical activity, xi, 1, 2, 4, 12, 23, 25, 26, 27,
    28, 29, 31, 33, 34, 38, 40, 46, 47, 48, 49
physical exercise, xi, 2, 4, 11, 19, 47
physical fitness, 26, 34, 35
placebo, 39
plasma, xi, 8, 12, 13, 14, 17, 18, 19, 20, 24,
    25, 26, 28, 36, 38, 41, 42, 44, 46
plasma levels, 9, 14, 28
plasminogen, 35
predictors, 33, 34
prevention, 29, 31, 33, 40
pro-atherogenic, 29
production, xi, 3, 4, 8, 9, 15, 17, 18, 19, 23,
    27, 28, 30, 31, 36, 39, 43, 44, 45, 48
program, 24, 26, 27, 28, 29
pro-inflammatory, xii, 3, 4, 9, 12, 13, 15, 17,
    18, 23, 27, 30
proteins, 3, 12, 18, 35
protocol, 20
psychosocial factors, 47
public health, 21

R

race, 25, 28
randomized controlled clinical trials, 25
receptors, 3, 18, 40
recovery, 12, 14
recurrence, 38
redistribution, 12
regeneration, 3, 7, 11, 36, 38
regulation, 15, 18, 29, 40, 41, 44

relationship, 9, 25, 26, 27, 34
relationships, 46
relevance, 27, 42
repair, 4
resistance, 2, 8, 14, 42, 47
respiratory, 25, 26, 37, 41
rheumatoid arthritis, 7, 8, 9, 23, 37, 39
risk, 1, 7, 9, 11, 12, 24, 26, 30, 35, 38, 39, 40, 46
risk factors, 1, 7, 26, 30, 35

S

safety, 35
sample, 48
sarcopenia, 7
sensitivity, 46
sepsis, 12
serum, 7, 15, 20, 24, 25, 26, 28, 47, 48, 49
sex, 20, 25, 28
signal transduction, 3, 8
skeletal muscle, 2, 3, 4, 7, 8, 14, 15, 17, 35, 36, 37, 38, 42, 43, 44, 46
skin, 9, 40
smokers, 26
smoking, 25
specificity, 44
sports, 34, 46
stability, 18
stabilization, 37
sterile, 7
strength, 15, 23, 25, 28
stress, 39, 43
successful aging, 46
suppression, 9, 19, 36
surveillance, 9
survival, 38
susceptibility, xi
symptoms, xi, 41
synthesis, 18

T

T cell, 43, 45

T lymphocytes, 4
TGF, 24
therapy, 35, 39
threshold, 21, 27
timing, 24
tissue, 3, 4, 8, 15, 25, 26, 39
TNF, 3, 4, 7, 8, 9, 12, 13, 17, 18, 19, 23, 27, 28, 37, 38, 43, 44, 45, 48
TNF-alpha, 38, 43, 44, 45
TNF-α, 3, 7, 8, 12, 13, 18, 19
total cholesterol, 27
training, 1, 11, 15, 23, 24, 25, 26, 27, 28, 29, 35, 42, 46, 47, 48, 49
training programs, 24, 25
transcription, 8, 18, 36, 44
transduction, 3, 19
transforming growth factor, 24, 36
trauma, 3
trial, 27, 35, 39, 47, 49
tumor, 3, 9, 37, 38, 40, 44, 45, 46
tumor necrosis factor, 3, 37, 38, 40, 44, 45, 46
turnover, 39
type 2 diabetes, xi, 1, 2, 7, 8, 9, 35, 38

U

ulcerative colitis, 9, 39, 40
upper respiratory tract, 41

V

values, 11
variability, 24
variables, 46
variation, 26, 42
vastus lateralis, 15
viral infection, 36
viruses, 4
vitamin C, 40
vitamins, 43

W

walking, 20, 26

weight loss, 25, 26, 29, 44, 48, 49
white blood cell count, 25
women, 25, 27, 28, 33, 34, 35, 47, 48

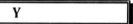

Y

young adults, 48
young women, 20